SYNTHESIS IN HEALING

Also by Judy Jacka

A Philosophy of Healing
A-Z of Natural Therapies
Meditation—The Most Natural Therapy
Healing Through Earth Energies
Frontiers of Natural Therapies
Healing Yourself Naturally
The Vivaxis Connection

SYNTHESIS IN HEALING

Subtle Energies *and* Natural Therapies for Optimal Health

Judy Jacka

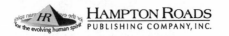

HAMPTON ROADS
PUBLISHING COMPANY, INC.

Cover design by Marjoram Productions
Cover art © 2003 M. Freeman/PhotoLink/Getty Images
Interior illustrations by Anne L. Louque

Hampton Roads Publishing Company, Inc.
1125 Stoney Ridge Road
Charlottesville, VA 22902

434-296-2772
fax: 434-296-5096
e-mail: hrpc@hrpub.com
www.hrpub.com

If you are unable to order this book from your local
bookseller, you may order directly from the publisher.
Call 1-800-766-8009, toll-free.

Library of Congress Cataloging-in-Publication Data
Jacka, Judy.
  Synthesis in healing : subtle energies and natural
therapies for optimal health / Judy Jacka.
      p. ; cm.
Includes bibliographical references and index.
  ISBN 1-57174-298-0 (alk. paper)
  1. Alternative medicine. 2. Holistic medicine. 3. Naturopathy.
  [DNLM: 1. Naturopathy—methods. 2. Holistic Health.
  3. Homeopathy methods. WB 935 J12s 2003] I. Title.
  R733.J24 2003
  615.5—dc21
2003001981

                    ISBN 1-57174-298-0
                    10 9 8 7 6 5 4 3 2 1
          Printed on acid-free paper in the United States

Dedication

This book is dedicated to both the memory and legacy of writings from Alice Bailey whose treatise, *Esoteric Healing*, has been a beacon for more than thirty years of my life; and to Brenda Johnston, who founded the International Network of Esoteric Healing and who is a pioneer of healing in the energy field.

Table of Contents

Foreword

This book on holistic healing is a gift to all of us from a well-respected and internationally renowned author, teacher, clinician and healer, Judy Jacka. It is a timely gift at this time as more and more people are combining conventional with alternative therapies and doing "spiritual questing" to attempt to understand the soul. This book is one of the first to offer concrete information about how to heal both the inner and the outer self.

Many best-selling books in the United States discuss healing from one perspective or another. Examples include *Anatomy of the Spirit* by Caroline Myss, *Miracle Cures: Dramatic New Scientific Discoveries Revealing Healing Powers of Herbs, Vitamins and other Natural Remedies* by Jean Carper, *Eating Well for Optimum Health* by Andrew Weil, and *The Seat of the Soul* by Gary Zukav. However, no book currently on the market combines all these perspectives. There seems to be a yearning for just the synthesis of inner and outer healing that Judy Jacka, an accomplished pioneer in naturopathic medicine, has provided.

Over the years, Judy Jacka has bridged natural therapies with medical science, developed an accredited curriculum in Australia, and explored other methods of healing. She has used these multiple modalities in working with clients in her clinics throughout Australia and has taught these techniques in seminars around the world. This book provides case studies of her clinical work and includes information about minerals, vitamins, herbs, homeopathy, flower essences, and bodywork, and provides clarity about the role of chakras and energy fields. Information on esoteric healing and the curriculum she developed for teaching this method of working with the soul are presented in an understandable and helpful manner. As the author states, "The quest for the soul becomes larger than the healing of the individual."

I feel fortunate to have studied with Judy Jacka over several years as she taught her new curriculum on esoteric healing. As her student, I learned how to deepen and focus my own spiritual life and healing ability. Her techniques were personally beneficial when I developed breast cancer. Even as a college professor in the Ivy League in the U.S. and at other prestigious universities, I learned some new and improved teaching techniques from her. Studying with her had a profound impact on my life and work.

I was also able to witness an example of Judy's own healing using a technique described in this book. While presenting a seminar at her Australian clinic, she emerged one spring morning with her eyes swollen and her throat affected from a severe allergic reaction to the blooms of the wattle trees. I was sure she would be unable to conduct our session that day. However, she walked outside and bathed her eyes with water treated on a selected energy location on her property. I have to admit, I had been quite skeptical the previous day when she explained Earth energies and showed me her Vivaxis techniques. My skepticism turned to amazement as she re-entered the clinic about ten minutes later. Her swollen eyes were now bright and open, her voice fully reinstated, and all signs of her allergic reaction had vanished. It was then that I also became a believer in this subject, which she described in *The Vivaxis Connection* (Hampton Roads, 2000), her previous book.

This new book is the result of more than three decades of Judy's teaching and learning about the human body and spirit. The author generously shares her knowledge and experience at a time when there is a new readiness to hear and learn about techniques that complement, supplement, and surpass what is known about healing through conventional medical wisdom. The book is clearly written without the jargon and hype that we tend to hear from many of the new age "gurus." The examples are clear and helpful. Her teaching techniques are superior, even when presented through the printed word. She combines her own rich experience and background with examples from scientists, philosophers, psychologists, other cultures, religious masters, and scientific studies.

This book is an important contribution to our understanding of how disease and pollution impact our bodies. While I wish it were required reading in every medical school, I know that some colleges may not be ready for this book. However, I am encouraged that some medical schools throughout the world are broadening their curriculum to include nutrition and other healing methods in their training of conventional doctors. Perhaps during the twenty-first century we will see the recognition of the healing of the soul and the body through the many techniques mentioned in this text. We are fortunate that Judy Jacka has blended the soul approach with natural therapies in her excellent new book.

—Cynthia S. Johnson, Ph.D.
Professor Emeritus, National Center for Higher Education,
California State University, Long Beach, California

Senior Scholar in Residence
American College Personnel Association
Washington, D.C.

Acknowledgments

As with all books containing unusual material I have been particularly concerned with gaining appropriate feedback and guidance for the various processes involved. I acknowledge and thank the contribution of the International Network of Esoteric Healing (INEH) for my training in this healing approach and also for many of the triangles described in the text including those on which the sketches are based.

In particular, I am grateful for the inspiration received from the writings of Alice Bailey via the Lucis Trust. These writings have always taken a pivotal place in my life, especially the teachings about healing. A number of the triangles developed in the practical work of the INEH are related to triangles mentioned in the Bailey literature.

Grateful thanks are offered to all those clients who permitted their case histories to be described. Some of the material is of a sensitive nature and without their consent and enthusiasm the book would not have been possible. I am very happy to have the Foreword written by my friend, professor Cynthia Johnson, who as an educator specializing now in spiritual values within education, is a most appropriate critic of the book.

My appreciation goes also to editor Richard Leviton, whose suggestions are sometimes challenging but always useful. Finally, my loving thanks to my life partner John Garretty, who read the manuscript as a lay person and who was thus able to make valuable suggestions to increase the reader's understanding.

Introduction

In this book, I present a synthesis of inner and outer healing. For thirty years, I have practiced as a natural therapist using a blend of vitamins, minerals, herbs, homeopathy, and flower essences plus a form of bodywork known as Bowen Therapy. This has proved to be an excellent approach for most physical conditions. Through re-educating clients about their nutrition and lifestyle, they have been able to maintain improvements in health after discontinuing naturopathic treatment. In addition, I have introduced clients to the deeper aspects of healing and the practice of meditation.

Throughout this time, I have studied and practiced meditation myself, and made a study of many philosophical and practical approaches to the more subtle aspects of disease. During the last ten years, I have included an esoteric approach that addresses the inner causes of health and disease. Since I started blending subtle healing with natural therapies, I have found that the treatment time is greatly shortened and there is a more lasting recovery for clients.

There are many approaches to medicine in traditional cultures that place a profound emphasis on inner factors in addition to the outer causes of disease. Examples are the medical approaches of the Australian Aborigines and American Indians, Tibetan and Chinese medicine, and to a certain extent, early Greek medicine. Early last century in Germany (and later, Switzerland), Rudolf Steiner pioneered a medical approach known as anthroposophical medicine. Doctors and therapists who use this approach acknowledge the importance of restoring balance to the energies underlying physical organs and also to the subtle energy fields associated with emotions and thoughts.

As you can see from figure 1, the early naturopaths in Europe placed some importance on the inner factors of thoughts and emotions on

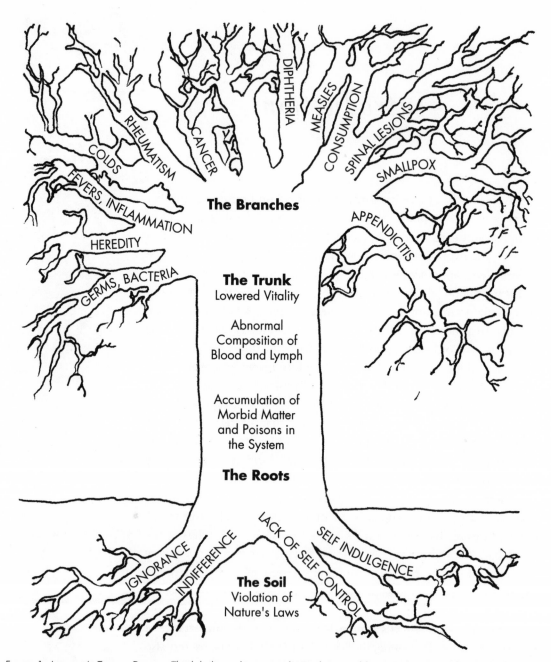

FIGURE 1: LINDLAHR'S TREE OF DISEASE. The labels on this tree indicate that in addition to the central focus of infections and toxins, Lindlahr labeled the roots to include factors relating to emotional and lifestyle issues.

disease. Unfortunately, the modern naturopathic movement has tended to ignore the inner causes of disease in an attempt to gain recognition and scientific acclaim for their physical therapies of vitamins, minerals, herbs, and homeopathic remedies. However, homeopathy in particular has always addressed the whole person, including one's emotional and mental characteristics.

More recently, psycho-neuro-immunology (PNI) has established beyond doubt the effect of the emotions and thoughts on our biochemistry. Even an actor playing a particular character can profoundly change their own blood picture, in terms of white cells and antibodies, in a few moments. Pioneers in PNI have started to work directly on the energy fields surrounding the body, in keeping with this emerging understanding of inner factors that influence health and disease.

Other pioneers of subtle energy therapy include nursing professor Doris Krieger, who has taught what she terms Therapeutic Touch to more than 30,000 nurses and doctors during the second half of the last century. Nurses further developed this science into a system known as Healing Touch, whereby the human energy field is examined and treated in more detail using the traditional chakra system. Barbara Brennan, a scientist and healer, has developed a training course for diagnosis and treatment using the chakras. The chakras are understood to be energy centers that underlie or sub-stand the main seven endocrine glands and their associated organs and tissues. Thus there are seven main endocrine glands and seven main chakras, which transmit our different levels of consciousness. She examines in detail the energy fields surrounding and underlying the physical body.

Over the last forty years, I have studied many approaches to healing in which the inner factors are added to the outer. In the more extreme New Age examples, "negative emotions" and thoughts are considered to be the only cause of disease, and affirmations are suggested for each situation. This approach sometimes totally ignores fairly obvious physical causes and has caused unnecessary guilt in some persons. Each therapist and teacher will obviously have some outstanding cases to justify the value of their particular therapeutic system, and obviously there is some validity in each approach.

Being pragmatic by nature, I am therefore interested in the greatest good for the greatest number of people. For this reason, I have steered clear of any extremes in my practice of healing. My early studies of Theosophy, anthroposophical medicine, and the teachings of Alice Bailey led me to her treatise *Esoteric Healing*. The term "esoteric" simply means subjective or inner healing—the use of techniques not normally recognized and accepted. I found the Bailey treatise to be the most profound, logical, and inspiring of all the approaches to healing I have studied over decades of searching.

Alice Bailey wrote 24 metaphysical books over a period of thirty years and these works were written under telepathic impression from a Tibetan teacher known as Djwhal Khul. Bailey was born in 1880 in Manchester, England, and began her spiritual journey as a young Christian evangelist during the First World War. After her first marriage to a protestant clergyman, she moved to the USA and after he died she began the journey into the teachings featured in her books. She also founded the Arcane School in 1919. To this day, the work of the Lucis Trust, which now runs the school, relies almost totally on donations apart from the sale of the books. The teaching on esoteric healing is one of many subjects, including cosmology, psychology, and astrology covered in the Bailey books.

From my perspective, the central tenet of the subtle aspect of healing is to invoke the healing essence or soul of the client. In this sense, the healer becomes a spiritual midwife who assists in invoking the soul of the client to flow through all levels of their energy field and finally through the physical body.

I discovered an international group that partly based their training program on the Bailey teachings. This group is known as the International Network of Esoteric Healers (INEH) and it began its international work in England. The INEH sent two teachers, at my request, in 1988 to Australia and for the next three years a group of Melbourne therapists studied and practiced their teachings. However, there was no written curriculum other than three pages of subject headings and a few diagrams. So after graduating from this course I designed a substantial curriculum. It included all the INEH subjects, but also many other central teachings of Alice Bailey about healing. Later, I was able to contribute to the curriculum eventually developed by the INEH.

The Bailey teachings on healing included a lot of instruction about the chakras decades before any other teachings on the subject were available. In particular, there is a treatise on psychology that places an emphasis on the soul or inner essence of the individual. Throughout the Bailey treatises there is instruction on how to align with the healing essence or soul energies so that these energies may sweep through the psyche and heal emotions and fragmented parts of the personality. Many physical health problems are considered to be caused by subjective disturbances of emotions and mind. However, the Bailey teachings on healing also stress the need for outer factors involving the physical body to be addressed, whether by the orthodox medical profession or complementary health therapists with appropriate training in medical sciences. Hence, my interest in combining natural therapies with esoteric healing.

After 1998, I started to integrate the principles of *Esoteric Healing* into my naturopathic practice, and now most of my clients receive this approach to energy balancing at each session. My basic practice of making a synthesis of minerals, vitamins, herbs, and homeopathy continues, but I now include healing in the energy field for most of my clients.

From my perspective, the central tenet of the subtle aspect of healing is to invoke the healing essence or soul of the client. In this sense, the healer becomes a spiritual midwife who assists in invoking the soul of the client to flow through all levels of their energy field and finally through the physical body. Without this process of centering, the client can become dependent on the healer, and there is the possibility of the "guru" scenario developing between client and therapist.

The use of natural therapies to remove toxins, increase vitality, and balance the biochemistry and nervous system forms the basis of treatment for my clients at the physical level. In *Synthesis in Healing*, I describe in detail both the inner and outer factors for health and disease according to my understanding. Then I describe the *modus operandi* of natural therapies and esoteric healing, after which I explore various categories of disease, both acute and chronic, for which a blend of subtle healing and natural therapies has produced a profound improvement in the client's health. This section includes numerous case histories.

The main aim of this book is to convey how, for lasting healing, we must have an understanding of both the inner and outer causes of disease. To demonstrate this, I present practical examples of how this has been achieved. Although I am not going to present a complete guide to either esoteric healing or natural therapies, exercises are included for you to develop your sense of healing touch and for working on your chakras and their possible associated physical disorders. For instance, digestive and reproductive exercises are included after the case histories on those topics. There are also detailed explanations of the naturopathic supplements prescribed for each case.

However, it is not my intention to give "cookbook" dosages for the remedies mentioned or for you to use this book for self-prescribing. You should seek out a well-qualified naturopath for that purpose. My intention is to give you understanding about the healing process on its inner and outer levels and how a synthesis in healing may lead to more profound levels of well-being.

PART ONE

1 The Outer Causes of Disease

Thirty years in clinical practice with more than 25,000 persons has convinced me that most disease has an inner and outer factor, although the proportion of each varies widely with each individual. For the purpose of this book, the outer will be designated as those factors in the physical environment of the individual that contribute to ill health. The physical environment in this model will include the physical body of the person and their inherited predispositions, plus their living and working environment.

In the last thirty years, there has been a much greater recognition on the part of the general public as to the outer causes of disease. Radio, television, and the Internet have been the means of spreading knowledge about health and disease. Indeed, surveys have revealed that programs about health and disease are the most popular of all non-fiction television programs. Since the 1980s, the health foods industry and its associated nutritional supplements industry have been the fastest growing industries, apart from computers. At least 60% of persons in the U.S. and Australia use nutritional supplements each year, and a large percentage of these persons consult a natural therapist at least once per year.[1] We will start with those environmental factors, the awareness of which first led the general public to realize that their bodies were a repository for harmful chemicals from the environment.

Environmental Pollution

Environmental pollution is the most generally recognized problem that contributes to our health problems, and was first highlighted

---

Table 1: Environmental and Chemical Pollution

Pharmaceutical drugs	Chemical pollution of drinking water
Lead from car exhausts	More than 5,000 chemical food additives
Acid rain from factory emissions	Environmental xeno-estrogens
Superphosphate and pesticides in foods	Electromagnetic pollution
Salinization of soils preventing farming	Mercury in tooth fillings
Formaldehyde inhalation from furnishings	

---

by Rachel Carson in the 1960s with her book *Silent Spring*.[2] Since then, governments have gradually become aware of and have made some attempt to pass legislation for the control of effluents from factories and other industrial sources. Even so, the burning of fossil fuels remains a controversial question among governments.

We still have enormous problems from chemical pollution in streams, rivers, and seas; high levels of lead in air in cities and towns; acid rain from factory emissions; and high levels of pesticides in some fruits, vegetables, and cereals. In addition, we are subject to thousands of chemicals added to foods for preserving, coloring, emulsifying, stabilizing, and disinfecting (see table 1).

In countries like Australia, there are also problems with the salinization of soils. This has been caused by unwise farming methods, whereby all the natural vegetation has been removed and the water table has gradually risen so that crops can no longer be grown on millions of acres formerly used for farming.

Poor Nutrition

Nutrition and the various components of our diet have come under scrutiny in relation to many health disorders. Books about health and nutrition have been published in perhaps greater numbers than on any other nonfiction subject. Even in airport bookshops the health section is almost as big as that of fiction. Poor nutrition probably still features as the most significant cause of outer disease. Thus some ethnic and national groups with poor educational and housing standards who have adopted the worst form of Western diets have greater infant mortality and higher rates of heart disease, diabetes, and other chronic diseases than Westerners.

Examples of these groups are the Aborigines in Australia, the Maoris in New Zealand, and Native Americans. It is interesting that these groups had their own successful forms of traditional medicine before adopting unhealthy Western lifestyles. Their deteriorating health could also be attributed to a loss of their own spiritual values as they strive to copy Westerners, the emphasis on owning cars and television sets, and the seeming addiction to the busyness, noise, and stress of life.

Dietary surveys of particular groups such as children and the elderly in the West have revealed that many persons are deficient in basic elements like calcium, magnesium, zinc, and vitamins A, B, C, and E.[3] There is so much reading material on this subject that I do not wish to devote much space to describing the various syndromes of illness that can result from these deficiencies. As we go through the various case histories later, I will give details of particular dietary needs.

Accumulation of Toxins

Apart from the many deficiencies and indeed in some cases, due to such deficiencies, toxins can accumulate in organs and connective tissues of the body. Examples of toxins that can accumulate in our bodies are mercury from dental amalgam fillings, pharmaceutical drugs, excess copper from water pipes, lead from exhaust fumes, petrochemical toxins, superphosphates from fertilizers, fungicides and insecticides in foodstuffs, fluoride in water supplies, cadmium in plastics, and formaldehyde from foam plastic in home furnishings.

I was interested to see on a television science show that some medical investigation suggests that toxins in the body's connective tissue can develop from an amalgamation of excess sugar in the body with protein to form a caramel-type substance that clogs the brain and body tissues. There is also a suggestion from biochemical sources that metals such as mercury and lead may combine with proteins to form plaques in brain tissue. Further research is obviously needed, but these factors could well be the basis for chronic fatigue syndrome (CFS) and perhaps Alzheimer's disease. It may account for the new toxic signs I have seen in the irises (by way of iridological analysis) of many persons over the last fifteen years. These signs appear as hundreds of almost microscopic dark brown dots scattered through the area of the iris that corresponds to connective tissue, according to iridology.

Basic naturopathic principles suggest that a poor diet with lots of refined sugar and foods high in cholesterol leads to a gradual accumulation of waste in the body that sooner or later manifests in lowered immunity and loss of energy. If the body has reasonable vitality, it may eliminate the waste by means of a fever and/or heavy mucous discharge. However, in most cases, the waste products gradually accumulate to manifest as chronic disease such as arthritis, asthma, chronic bronchitis, cancer, multiple sclerosis, severe exhaustion, and chronic fatigue syndrome.

Prescription Drugs

Periodically, current affairs programs highlight the percentage of hospital admissions that are caused by bad effects from prescribed doses of pharmaceutical drugs. In addition, we need to consider those medications that are freely available over the counter. A few years ago, a popular science program in Australia highlighted a medical article that claimed the most popular asthma drug had serious side effects and could be responsible for asthma deaths. There was a temporary public furor (one in four Australian children suffer from asthma) and then total silence on the matter. All public debate was silenced. Was this silence because drug companies have a very powerful control on orthodox medicine and the media?

There is certainly more awareness by the public of the side effects of pharmaceutical drugs, and this is one of the reasons why natural therapies became popular. People became aware that just as the external environment was becoming polluted, their internal environment or body was similarly becoming polluted. Chemicals prescribed by doctors have to be seen as a leading "outer" cause of disease. The immediate symptoms of a health problem may disappear or become suppressed with drugs, but the underlying causes are not addressed or resolved, so the drugs actually *contribute* to chronic disease.

The overuse of drugs is an aspect of physician-caused disease, known as iatrogenic disease.[4] One outstanding example is the overuse of antibiotics for both humans and livestock with the result that we are now faced with "super-germs" that are resistant to nearly all known antibiotics. This is another major reason why people have turned to natural remedies to improve their immunity to viruses and bacteria.

Inherited Factors and Predispositions

We have predispositions to certain chronic diseases. There is no doubt that a *tendency* to asthma, arthritis, and certain forms of cancer sometimes has a genetic basis. Often these tendencies can be side-stepped and their manifestation eliminated by a good diet, the use of certain nutritional supplements and, in particular, homeopathic remedies. Homeopathy calls these inherited tendencies miasms, and a skilled homeopath can help to eliminate them from your family lineage.

Inherited factors will also be strongly conditioned by those inner factors that relate to our emotions and thoughts. We will study this later, when looking at the inner factors. There are obviously some purely genetic factors, such as diseases like hemophilia. In this disease, hemorrhage from even small cuts can occur. Another example is thalassemia, a genetic condition that occurs in some Mediterranean people, causing serious anemia that does not permanently respond to treatment. However, many inherited tendencies are triggered as a result of poor lifestyle. Late onset diabetes (usually Type II) is a good example of an inherited tendency that in Australia has reached plague proportions, due chiefly to obesity and poor diet. Most likely, as the U.S. has a similar obesity problem amongst its population, the same increase will be observed.

Electromagnetic Pollution

Health problems from exposure to electromagnetic fields have only recently been recognized by more than a few concerned scientists.

Communities have started to challenge authorities intending to erect phone towers next to homes and children's playgrounds. Real estate agents have noted over the last few years that people are less likely to purchase a home near overhead high voltage power cables. The general public is also now aware that a certain amount of electromagnetic radiation is received by users of computers, television sets, and mobile and cell phones.

Studies have indicated that headaches, depression, and suicide are more common in persons living close to high voltage transmission lines. These problems are related to what is known as extremely low frequency (ELF) electromagnetic fields. The use of electric blankets and water beds has been shown to reduce factors in the blood related to immunity. High frequency fields include microwaves, and these can be encountered from mobile phones and their towers and also from leaking microwave ovens.

It is probably not any one factor that we should consider here, in relation to electromagnetic pollution, but the sum of our daily exposure. This may include time spent at the computer, exposure to television if sitting near the set, use of mobile phones, hair dryers, electric blankets, exposure to digital clocks near the head of the bed, leaking microwave ovens, and proximity to overhead power lines.[5]

The basic reason why these electromagnetic fields affect us adversely relates to the overriding effect they have on our own electromagnetic fields. Our human fields are very delicate compared to the fields created by modern technology. Our electromagnetic field is intimately connected with immunity, so if it is impaired we are more susceptible to infections and chronic disease such as cancer. No one would wish to go back to the days before technology; however, by understanding electromagnetic effects, we can plan our lives so as to minimize our contact with human-made electromagnetic fields. We can also boost our immunity with the use of antioxidants such as vitamins C and E.

X rays are another potent cause of problems from a high frequency source. This form of diagnosis is obviously essential in modern medicine, but it has the effect of disturbing all the carbon and calcium atoms in our bones, and this effect can be permanent. I have described this problem in detail in a previous book (*The Vivaxis Connection*, Hampton Roads, 2000), including a simple way to eradicate the negative effects of X rays. Mammograms and computerized temography (CT scans) are in the same category, and the radiation received from them is greater than from X-rays. These exposures all have a profound effect on the human energy field.

Summary: The outer causes of disease are many and include environmental pollution involving chemicals that pollute food, water, air, and earth; poor nutrition, which is partly due to deficiencies in food from poor farming methods and partly due to poor diet; inherited factors that affect metabolism; accumulation of toxins from an inability of the body to metabolize or eliminate waste products adequately through the normal channels of bowel, kidneys, skin, and lungs; overuse of prescription and over-the-counter drugs; and electromagnetic pollution from man-made sources such as high voltage transmission lines, mobile phones and towers, computer and television screens, water beds, and electric blankets.

2 A Synthesis of Therapies for Physical Problems

When treating the physical body, I have found a synthesis of therapies to be the most effective. In particular, the outer causes of diseases are so numerous that only a carefully selected combination of vitamins, minerals, herbs, and homeopathy seem to resolve current physical ailments. Occasionally, this approach needs to be married with pharmaceutical drugs as prescribed by an orthodox practitioner. Examples of when conventional drugs may need to be continued are heart problems, blood pressure, and severe forms of asthma.

There are now more than 100 natural therapies in the Western world and an equal number of training programs although many of these have no accreditation. In my practice, I have found that the traditional therapies of clinical nutrition, including the use of vitamins and minerals, herbal medicine, homeopathy, and a simple form of body work based on "trigger" points called Bowen Therapy, answer the needs of most clients, at the physical level. The inner factors will be addressed in the next chapter. Apart from Bowen Therapy, each of these modalities has a long history of clinical application, and clinical trials in these areas are at last beginning. Most of the current scientific research is focused on vitamins, minerals, and herbs, and not so much on homeopathy.

Due to the special qualities of whole herbs and homeopathic remedies some positive changes can take place in the psyche of the client who uses them. Therefore, to some extent, it is arbitrary to separate these external therapeutic approaches from more subtle inner healing therapies. Each physical therapy, whether minerals, vitamins, herbs, homeopathy, or bodywork, has its own sphere of action, although these spheres tend to overlap. For the understanding of the reader, it will be useful to briefly describe the nature and sphere of action for each modality mentioned so that when we get to the practical cases you will have a basic understanding of these therapies.

Minerals—The Basic Building Blocks

The twelve tissue salts are based on minerals that are essential for health. They were pioneered by Dr. W. H. Schuessler of Oldenburg, Germany, who first published articles on the tissue salts in 1873. He wrote that the structure and function of our organs depends upon the presence of finely balanced quantities of inorganic constituents. His written work went through 56 editions and was translated into many languages. Schuessler died in 1898.[6] Since that time, therapists have used the tissue salts in colloidal form for many health disorders. A colloid is a very fine suspension of particles—the form in which plants assimilate minerals from the soil; they are suspended in colloidal form within the water taken up by the roots.

Humans and animals assimilate minerals more adequately in colloidal form. When I first went into clinical practice, there was only one Australian firm that produced colloidal supplements with any quantifiable level of minerals—Blackmore's. Due to the high levels of deficiencies in some of the basic minerals, Maurice Blackmore developed his colloidal minerals to contain much higher levels of the mineral salts than were present in the traditional tissue salts. Practitioners in Australia who started using his "celloids" in the 1960s began obtaining much quicker and lasting rates of recovery in their clients. However, celloids are not available in all countries, and in the U.S., the Schuessler tissue salts should be substituted.

You will note when reading the case histories later in the book that I frequently refer to minerals in colloidal form. Apart from the celloids and Schuessler tissue salts, liquid varieties of colloidal minerals are available. Since the 1990s, a number of companies have been alerting the general public to the need for minerals in colloidal form.

Many companies sell minerals that are not in colloidal form, and some of the combinations are not appropriate for human medication. An example is a mixture of calcium and magnesium carbonate or "dolomite." These salts can only be absorbed if a person has a lot of hydrochloric acid in the stomach. I remember a client who came to our clinic after taking dolomite for many months; he had bladder stones. When analyzed, the chemical composition of the stones was in exactly the same proportion as the calcium and magnesium carbonate he had consumed as dolomite.

Minerals needed for our health include iron, calcium, magnesium, zinc, copper, phosphorous, sodium, sulfur, potassium, and silica, but we also need trace amounts of elements like chromium, fluoride, manganese, selenium, vanadium, and germanium. Large amounts of the last six minerals can be toxic. Examples of other common toxic elements in our environment include some heavy metals such as mercury, aluminum, lead, and cadmium.

During the twentieth century, farming methods changed drastically and the practice of crop rotation generally ceased. The land was forced to constantly produce more with the aid of super phosphates; at the same time, the use of toxic insecticides and fungicides became common. Chemical analysis of grains, cereals, and vegetables revealed a drop of up to 30-50% in mineral levels from crops grown in the second half of the twentieth century. Widespread mineral deficiencies therefore developed throughout the human population.[7]

Another reason for mineral deficiencies in our bodies is the increased intake of refined foods, in particular, white flour and sugar found in most packaged and canned foods available at supermarkets. I find it interesting when treating Asian people who come from rice-producing countries that they are initially horrified when I suggest that they should eat *brown* rice. For decades, they have copied the Western habit of refining grains and they now consider "brown" rice to be food for peasants and only white rice to be fit to eat.

There is also the prevalent use of pasta as the main evening meal. This means that the major part of the meal consists of refined flour. It also means that the daily vegetable intake is substantially reduced due the substitution of pasta for the traditional three vegetables. Instead, there is perhaps only a sauce consisting of a few finely chopped vegetables, garlic, flavoring, plus meat or fish pieces. The old standard meal of protein and three vegetables has disappeared in many family dietary regimens except for a couple times per week. Many of my clients have pasta three to four times a week, or more, so

I encourage them to at least use wholemeal pasta and to accompany it with a fresh green salad.

The use of white sugar in most biscuits, cakes, pastries, drinks, and sweets is one of the major causes of the extraordinary obesity problem in America and Australia (at least 50% of Australians are overweight). As a result of this sugar intake, Type II diabetes, which used to be *late*-onset, is now frequently affecting younger persons. A deficiency of the trace mineral chromium can cause sugar craving. Ironically, chromium is found in the unrefined extract from sugar-cane called molasses. The use of blackstrap molasses in the diet is a rich source of many minerals including potassium, magnesium, zinc, and chromium. One tablespoon per day is a good amount to use; it can be dissolved in hot water for convenient use.

Other reasons for mineral deficiencies relate to the antagonizing effect from heavy metals like lead and mercury. These metals displace calcium, magnesium, and zinc from the body. Some populations are exposed to high levels of lead from exhaust fumes in large cities and towns. Most people who had dental work undertaken in the twentieth century have amalgam fillings in their teeth, and these fillings contain mercury. The mercury gradually leeches out of the fillings due to the acids in foods and from aging fillings, and it is often then stored in body organs such as the thyroid, heart, and kidneys.

Levels of this toxic element and others can be established with blood and hair analysis. There are a number of nontoxic preparations such as antioxidants, the herb coriander, and other substances such as lipoic acid that can safely remove these substances from the body.

Inherited predispositions (homeopathy's miasms) are a further factor causing mineral problems. For example, someone in your family tree four generations ago may have suffered tuberculosis which then appears to cause a lack of calcium assimilation in later generations, such as yours. The main reason given in homeopathic literature for this lack of calcium assimilation is related to the slight disturbances in the physiology of some family members whose forbears suffered from tuberculosis. For this reason, resolution of residual bronchial problems and chest weakness is achieved by taking the tissue salt calcium phosphate.

Other predispositions to mineral imbalance stem from the presence of syphilis in the family tree. We are reminded of the biblical injunction—"the sins of the forefathers will be visited on us unto the fourth generation." There are not many families exempt from some degree of inherited predispositions or miasms. Homeopaths have specialized in understanding these inherited tendencies and have found that these taints can be eradicated with the use of homeopathy by a skilled practitioner. The use of homeopathy will be discussed shortly.

Generally, I find in clinical practice that it takes six months of mineral therapy for a deficiency to be corrected. But this resolution of the case will also depend on the lifestyle of the client. The stress of modern living and work can often mean that the tissue salts for the nervous system, such as magnesium and potassium phosphate, need constant replenishment.

Generally, I find in clinical practice that it takes six months of mineral therapy for a deficiency to be corrected. But this resolution of the case will also depend on the lifestyle of the client. The stress of modern living and work can often mean that the tissue salts for the nervous system, such as magnesium and potassium phosphate, need constant replenishment. Thus, the continuing use of these salts can be considered a form of health insurance.

Some minerals have a synergistic action with other elements or substances while others have an antagonistic effect. For this reason, self-prescribing without considerable study is not always a good idea. For instance, many calcium compounds are antagonistic to magnesium, a mineral needed for over fifty enzyme chains in the body. The modern obsession with preventing the development of osteoporosis has resulted in many women taking calcium supplements that are poorly assimilated. These may worsen arthritis, increase tendency to kidney stones or heel spurs, and may cause a magnesium deficiency.

Another example of unwise self-prescribing relates to individuals taking zinc for no particular reason. Zinc is antagonistic to copper, an element needed for healthy red blood cells. Other synergistic effects are found in the assimilation of iron, which is greatly increased when accompanied by vitamin C.

If you do not consult with a well-trained natural therapist then you should study one of the hundreds of well-written books on vitamins and minerals before self-prescribing.[8] Most manufacturing companies have self-help lines although these will obviously be biased towards their own products.

Vitamins—The Catalysts

The use of vitamins in clinical practice only dates back to the 1950s, although we can reflect that sailors in earlier times were given lemon and lime juice to prevent the vitamin C deficiency disease known as scurvy. Other discoveries along these lines led to the prevention of beriberi and the unpleasant skin disorder pellagra. Both these conditions were found to be helped by the use of brown rice, which is rich in B vitamins. The isolation and manufacture of the various vitamins belongs to the twentieth century, and most research occurred from the second half of the twentieth century onwards. Although this is not a textbook for vitamin therapy, there are some overall considerations worth mentioning.

Vitamins act as catalysts in the body for biochemical processes. They provide the energy for many reactions in the body and are used up in the process. They are also synergistic among themselves so that vitamin E works better in the presence of vitamin A. Some vitamins are destroyed by medical drugs, such as the vitamin B complex by the contraceptive pill. Heavy metals such as lead, mercury, and cadmium use up vitamin C reserves and displace essential minerals.

Dietitians often tell people they should be able to get enough vitamins from their food if it is well chosen, but medical surveys have revealed that people are often short on various vitamins. Otherwise, why would pregnant women be advised by orthodox doctors to take the B complex component called folic acid to prevent spina bifida in their unborn child? (Spina bifida is a congenital malformation of the spine.) The recommended daily allowance (RDA) of vitamins does not take into account the stress of twenty-first-century living. For instance, we need a good and constant supply of vitamin B complex to prevent stress and depression and to give us the energy and ability to concentrate. B complex is a water-soluble vitamin, so it is quickly excreted in the urine and needs to be replenished daily.

The other water-soluble vitamin needed in large quantities to prevent stress and to boost the immune function and prevent infection is vitamin C. Due to the way fruits and vegetables are stored today, vitamin C is largely deficient in all our foods unless home grown and eaten shortly after picking. It is completely destroyed in all cooking and heating processes and is oxidized almost immediately after cutting the fruit as the oxygen in the air destroys the vitamin C. Most people can do with a gram (1,000 mg) of vitamin C per day, but individual requirements vary enormously. During the stress of infection such as a flu virus, we often need up to eight or ten grams (8,000 or 10,000 mg) daily for a few days.

This brings me to discuss natural versus synthetic vitamins. While it would be ideal to have vitamins in their completely natural form from food, this is not practical for the large amounts we need today. The only vitamin we could obtain in large amounts from natural sources is vitamin D and this is actually toxic in large amounts. Hence, we don't eat polar bear liver even though it's high in vitamin D. To get sufficient vitamin B complex and vitamin C, it is usually necessary to take synthetic products. The same applies to the fat soluble vitamin E. In my years of clinical practice, I have never found any serious side effects in my clients from the use of synthetic vitamins. When you think of all the potentially harmful chemicals we imbibe in our food and water, it is illogical for purists to criticize the use of synthetic vitamins.

However, there is a lot of poor prescribing of vitamin products. For instance, many people take far too much vitamin B complex for their needs and can become hyperactive and perhaps insomniac as a result. Occasionally, a person is hypersensitive to the "fillers" in tablets and will get a skin rash or, in the case of the acid form of vitamin C, they may suffer slight inflammation of the stomach lining. The answer in this case is to take a buffered form of vitamin C or, if the problem is only mild, to have it after a meal.

We lose most of our water-soluble vitamins in the heating processes and cooking water. The fat-soluble vitamins A, D, and E are not lost so easily; as these vitamins are fat soluble, they can accumulate in the system. For this reason, vitamin A is now given in the form of beta-carotene. Occasionally I have a client whose skin has turned yellow because they have drunk too much carrot juice, but this soon disappears after reducing carrot intake, and no lasting harm is done.

Vitamin E is found in seeds, the kernels of nuts, and the germ of cereals. It oxidizes very easily, and the oil containing it becomes rancid.

For this reason capsules tend to be made from synthetic forms, and for any capsule containing oil it is essential to have a very good manufacturing process. Inexpensive versions of vitamin E should perhaps be avoided; the same applies to fish oil in capsules.

Refining of foods causes an almost complete loss of vitamins, so people on a diet that includes lots of refined sugar and flour are deficient in both minerals and vitamins. When I treat someone over a few months for a health disorder, I gradually introduce dietary changes so that when the treatment is tapered off their diet can largely take over as the therapy. However, for health insurance purposes, we should probably always include extra vitamins C and E for their antioxidant value.

An antioxidant prevents the accumulation of free radicals in our bodies. Free radicals are produced by our exposure to oxygen and to other more dangerous chemicals in the environment. Free radicals are chemical entities that damage the fatty membrane of cells and thus allow foreign invaders like virus and bacteria to enter the body. Harmful cell mutation, as in cancer, can occur more easily in the presence of free radicals. Over the last few years, many other valuable antioxidant agents have been discovered in addition to vitamin C and E; these include the Indian spice turmeric, green and black tea, grapeseed extract, and olive leaf extract.

Herbs—Stimulators of Function

Treatment of illness with herbs features in the history of most cultures and nations. Archeologists and historians have discovered evidence of botanic or herbal medicine in ancient Egypt, China, India, the Americas, and amongst the Aboriginal community in Australia. European herbs have been the subject of detailed research and application in the West.

Over the last few decades, considerable research and clinical trials have taken place, using herbs for medical conditions such as high blood pressure, diabetes, prostate disease, heart disease, and depression. A major sociological problem arises from the fact that most research is promoted and funded by drug companies who cannot patent naturally occurring herbs. This means that there is a tendency to take out the active principle of the herb and synthesize it so it can be patented.

Herbalists have always understood that the value in herbal medicine comes from the fact that the plant contains a balance of the active and supporting ingredients, thus minimizing and usually preventing the possibility of side effects. However, when the active ingredient is removed and concentrated, considerable side effects can be experienced, as is the case in many pharmaceutical products.

There are some herbs that need to be handled with care and given in only small doses such as the emetic lobelia, the abortifacient black cohosh, and the cardiac-specific foxglove. Well-trained herbalists are well aware of these parameters, and if you reflect on the level of hospital admissions and deaths due to complications from pharmaceutical drugs, the few cautions needed with respect to herbs and the few complaints reported from the use of herbal medicine are insignificant.

Herbs contain minerals, vitamins, enzymes, and subtle vitalizing components that seem to be common to plants in general.[9] They are a most suitable medication for most of our ills. Herbs are particularly useful for toning organs and improving their physiology. Part of this toning effect is due to their capacity to eliminate waste through the normal channels of bowel, kidneys, lungs, and skin. Herbs often have an affinity for particular parts of the body: for instance, dandelion or centaury for the liver; red clover and clivers for the lymphatic system; hops, oat seed, and passion flower for the nervous system. The usable parts of the herb vary, and can be the fruit, leaves, stem, or roots, depending on the type of herb and its medicinal use.

Herbs can be prescribed in liquids, teas, tablets, capsules, and powders, but I prefer using herbs in liquid form. For some reason, clients notice that the liquid form seems more effective. It probably has something to do with the ability of a liquid to be imprinted with the energy of the herbs. This quality can change the surface tension of the water molecules in our body after contact with the herb, so perhaps the more subtle effect of herbs may be better transmitted in liquid form. Some people cannot tolerate the fairly high percentage of medicinal alcohol in liquid herbs, while others cannot bear the taste of herbs or need tablets for convenience when traveling.

Manufacturing companies are constantly improving their extraction procedures, and this allows for increasingly purer preparations of the plant. Most Western countries now have very strict guidelines for the preparation of herbal substances, both in terms of farming procedures and manufacturing. Quality control is strictly monitored as in drug companies. The majority of colleges that train practitioners in herbal medicine now give a grounding in chemistry, biochemistry, and herbal medicine, as well as instruction in the art of treatment using a blend of four or five herbs to cover the needs of any particular person. The use of liquid herbs allows the therapist to make up an individual mixture for each person.

Homeopathy—Transformations with Miniscule Doses

The science and art of homeopathy is even more specialized than the practice of herbal medicine. Samuel Hahnemann (1755-1843), a medical doctor in Germany, pioneered this therapy, although there is evidence that the minute doses that characterize homeopathy were used earlier in some cultures.

The philosophy of homeopathy rests on the principle that "like cures like," also called the Doctrine of Similars. For instance, the symptoms of arsenic poisoning may be removed by giving a very high dilution of arsenic—high enough so that there are no physical molecules left in the remedy. Hahnemann began his career as a translator of chemical texts and when writing about cinchona bark, he disagreed with the findings reported, so he began to experiment on himself with the bark. He found that he developed shivering and fever, symptoms for which cinchona was normally prescribed to cure. Later he called this phenomenon the "proving" of the drug. To eliminate the side effects, Hahnemann reduced the dose and found that in *minute* doses, the drug was effective to treat malaria.

Thus began a long career in which Hahnemann painstakingly researched hundreds of substances and tested them on his students and disciples. He made detailed recordings on each substance he tested so that a comprehensive body of knowledge accumulated which was increased later by the research of other homeopaths, including the Americans James Kent and Constance Hering.

Homeopathic remedies may be prepared from mineral, plant, or animal substances. There are two main types of dilutions used—decimal and centesimal. In the case of the decimal system, one part of the substance is mixed with nine parts of the carrying medium—water or lactose—and thoroughly mixed or succussed (shaken). Then one part of that mixture is further diluted with another nine parts of the medium used and shaken again. This process is continued for the required number of dilutions. In the centesimal system, dilutions are based on 100 parts instead of ten. After about the thirtieth dilution, there are no physical molecules left.

The discovery that a particular number of dilutions removes all chemical molecules was made by the Italian physicist and chemist Amadeo Avogadro (1776–1856), and this finding is called Avogadro's number. It appears that the pattern of the remedy is present in the diluted medium and that this patterned substance can be used to treat the patient.

It can be imagined, therefore, that homeopathy is a very safe system and most suitable for persons who cannot tolerate large quantities of pills or strong-tasting herbal mixtures. It is particularly useful for treating the deep constitutional aspects of the person and for eradicating the inherited predispositions that Hahnemann researched.[10] These inherited tendencies are not usually resolved using herbs, and often need very high dilutions of homeopathic remedies, because doses at these strengths penetrate very deeply into the genetic makeup of the person.

Homeopathic remedies in low potencies such as six or twelve dilutions still have some chemical molecules and are most suitable for toning organs in the same way as herbs. In addition, homeopathy is an inexpensive form of medication for obvious reasons; the quantity of substance used is minute and the manufacturing process is very simple. There has not been as much research on homeopathy as on herbal medicine, but it is gradually increasing.

When constitutional prescribing is used a very detailed case history is taken, including all the idiosyncrasies of the client's physical, emotional, and mental life. This history is recorded so as to find a close match between the homeopathic remedy and the disease process. The homeopath therefore often becomes a very skilled psychologist. The patient history is often very important in chronic cases. The homeopath must not only choose one out of thousands of remedies, but must also choose the right potency. When these two criteria are fulfilled, the disease process is shattered as in the example of when a person sings a note that resonates with a glass and the glass breaks.

Homeopathy is therefore based on the principle of finding a sympathetic resonance between the disease process and the remedy. Readers will remember hearing how when soldiers cross a bridge they break step in case their marching rhythm causes the bridge to collapse because their marching rhythm may be in resonance with the vibratory rate of the bridge.

The homeopath must also know how to moderate the treatment so that there is not too sharp an aggravation for a couple of days when the dissolution of the disease process takes place. In the case of low potency homeopathy, there is much less likely to be a sharp aggravation. The lower potencies can be self-prescribed in some cases for acute problems like bee stings, colds, diarrhea, gastric upsets, ear infections, and other short-lived problems.

Homeopaths would regard this type of prescribing as symptomatic, but it can be relatively permanent if not complicated by inherited predispositions. Often a therapist will use a number of homeopathic remedies, both in high and low potencies, to cover every aspect of the case. For instance, she might prescribe remedies for toning the liver and lymphatic system while at the same time giving deep-acting remedies to resolve a tendency for warts or herpes.

Flower Essences

The first well-known system of flower essences was pioneered by a Harley Street physician, Edward Bach, early in the last century in England. Bach selected thirty-eight English wildflowers and flowering trees to treat a range of emotional diseases. The blossoms are picked from their wild state and soaked in glass containers exposed to the sun for some hours. The liquid is then strained and cask brandy used as a preservative. The stock is further diluted for purposes of prescribing.[11]

Examples of these remedies are Holly for jealousy, Willow for resentment, Vervain for stress, White Chestnut for persistent unwanted thoughts, Larch for confidence, and Cherry Plum for desperation. Five drops in water are administered orally at least three times daily, and more often in cases of trauma. The Bach flowers are very safe remedies because the remedy simply consists of the water in which the flower is soaked. The water appears to become imprinted with the quality and resonance of the flower, which is believed to be able to resolve emotional conditions.

Other systems for collecting flower potencies have been used. I once ran a workshop at my Melbourne home for a therapist who had pioneered some Australian remedies. All she did was put herself into a meditative state and drip water over the flowers on the plant and into a bottle! We did not find that the essences prepared in this way kept their potency. During the last two decades the line called Australian Bush essences have become very popular and widely used. There is an idea that the flowers growing in the client's own country are the most appropriate for treatment. However, I have found the English wildflowers give very good results, despite the fact that nearly 50% of the Australian population comes from countries other than the United Kingdom. Perhaps the Aboriginal people would respond best to Australian essences.

The California Flower Essence Society essences are also respected and widely used. The pioneers of these American wildflower-based essences were the first to talk about the application of flower essences for spiritual growth and treatment of the energy field and energy centers or chakras (see chapter 4). I have found that the chakras respond immediately to flower essences, and this is especially useful for people in shock. I often mix the flower essences with low potency homeopathic remedies, as you will note in some of the case histories.

Bodywork—The Universal Favorite

Healing is related to touch, and perhaps that is why bodywork is so popular. There are many kinds of bodywork that can be blended with the internal natural therapies. Popular examples are chiropractic, osteopathy, massage, acupressure, lymphatic drainage, shiatsu, and Bowen Therapy.

I have chosen in my practice to use Bowen Therapy, involving trigger points on the muscle fascia, because it is quick, painless, noninvasive, and it gives excellent and lasting results. An Australian named Tom Bowen pioneered this therapy in the 1940s, but we have very little information on how he developed the techniques. The trigger points are mostly in the position of acupuncture points, and the muscle covering in these areas is "rolled" over the points. Such techniques are now taught worldwide and have become particularly popular in Australia, New Zealand, and America.

Bodywork makes us feel good immediately, it improves blood and nerve supply, and stimulates lymphatic drainage. It thus assists the activities of oral remedies given to the client. From my perspective, bodywork is not as important as the internal therapies, provided a client gets a reasonable amount of exercise. But for the person who has chronic back or muscle problems, bodywork may be the chosen as the main line of treatment.

Synthesis in Prescribing

The emphasis in my practice has not been bodywork but making a synthesis of clinical nutrition, using vitamins and minerals, herbs, homeopathy, flower essences, and subtle energy healing (esoteric healing). I have found that, for some reason, synthesis is a difficult process to teach. Only a few natural therapists seem to master the art, and most tend to specialize in herbs, homeopathy, bodywork nutrition, or whatever. Even before adding the subtle treatment with esoteric healing as described in chapter 4, I find that making a synthesis of vitamins, minerals, herbs, and homeopathy produces excellent results with most disorders.

Perhaps it takes a certain kind of mind to be able to take in the information necessary for this task of synthesis, but the results are worth the effort. However, making a synthesis is more than having a repertory of minerals, vitamins, herbs, and homeopathy. The computer can do this task for us now. The art lies in perceiving the exact selection and emphasis needed for each individual. An example will clarify this.

Let us imagine that Jane has visited my clinic and describes how she is very tired even after a long sleep. Perhaps she has a persistent

The emphasis in my practice is making a synthesis of clinical nutrition, using vitamins and minerals, herbs, homeopathy, flower essences, and subtle energy healing (esoteric healing). Even before adding the subtle treatment with esoteric healing, I find that making a synthesis of vitamins, minerals, herbs, and homeopathy produces excellent results with most disorders.

and itchy rash on her legs; her periods are heavy and painful; and she suffers bad headaches just before menstruation. She is a computer programmer and can only exercise a little on weekends because her hours at work are so long. Her diet consists of a muffin and coffee for breakfast, salad and white roll for lunch, accompanied by an apple, and stir-fry vegetables and chicken or pasta for dinner at 8 P.M. Does this sound familiar?

From my perspective, Jane is obviously deficient in vitamin B complex and the tissue salts magnesium and potassium phosphate because these are all essential for energy and the nervous system. Her diet and symptoms of tiredness and headaches tell me about these deficiencies, even without any other examination. Painful periods can also relate to this mineral imbalance. Her diet and leg rash indicate that the lymphatic system is sluggish, and this may well be confirmed by signs in the iris.

She will therefore be given an herbal mixture with cleansing herbs like clivers, red clover, catmint, and burdock. In addition, homeopathic liver and lymphatic toning drops will be given with a few drops of the Bach flowers Cherry Plum for desperation and Hornbeam for strength. Finally, vitamin C will be prescribed to help detoxify the body because Jane does not have enough fruit or other raw food in her diet.

Over a few months, she will be educated in her diet to start the day with raw fruit to "wake up" her digestive enzymes; she will be urged to use wholemeal wheat or rye bread and wholemeal pasta to include more B complex in her diet and have a fresh salad at lunch time whenever possible. I would perhaps combine a Bowen treatment with the esoteric healing to balance her chakras and invoke the healing energies of the soul (described in detail later). With this sort of case, about 90% of persons have considerable improvement in the first month of treatment. Even if all their symptoms disappear during that time, it is suggested they consolidate their improvement with further months of treatments, particularly as the mineral deficiencies can take six months to resolve.

The next chapter will explore some of the inner causes of disease. Sometimes it is difficult to separate the inner from the outer, or rather, to establish which comes first, the chicken or the egg. This is especially the case in respect to choice of foods. For example, when people are depressed, they often turn to junk food like chocolate and milkshakes for comfort. But are they depressed because they are deficient in vitamin B complex and certain minerals, or does their depression cause them to choose a diet of junk food for a quick lift?

Summary: Minerals are the basic building blocks of the cells and are best assimilated in colloidal form because the particles are then very small and easily absorbed. The twelve tissue salts have been used for over one hundred years for this purpose, although there are other trace elements, such as chromium and zinc, which are very important. Vitamins act as catalysts for various biochemical processes and during disease processes are often needed in larger amounts than is present in our diets. They are easily lost by refining food and in cooking processes.

Herbs are also rich in trace elements, minerals, and enzymes, and have an extra life-giving factor that makes them peculiarly suitable to promote function of organs and tissues. Homeopathic remedies can be based on minerals, herbs, or animal tissue, and are able to penetrate very deeply, due to the diluting and shaking process during their manufacture. They are also able to resolve inherited tendencies to various diseases, due to their penetrative power. Due to the diluting and shaking process, they have a unique characteristic that has been coined as "like cures like."

Flower essences are another very subtle form of treatment used to treat many different negative emotional states and are also used to stimulate personality and spiritual growth. They are especially safe to use, as they have absolutely no side effects or even temporary aggravation.

A synthesis of these internal remedies can be married to a form of bodywork such as Bowen Therapy and/or combined with esoteric healing, which balances the chakras and invokes the healing energies of the soul.

3 The Inner Causes
of Disease

If the average person were asked what they think about the inner factors of disease, they would probably answer they are negative emotions like anger and depression. The public has had exposure to this concept because so many books and workshops have been developed over the last fifty years to highlight these factors. From my perspective, however, the inner causes of disease have a complexity that I will highlight in this chapter.

Contacting Our Healing Essence

A major theme in this book is the need to contact our healing essence or soul, by whatever name it is called. By contacting our essence, I mean having a transcendent experience that can be a tangible level of conscious functioning, even though it's beyond emotions, feelings, and thoughts. Such experiences were first mentioned in a clinical sense by the psychologist Abraham Maslow as "peak experiences," although foreshadowed by writers in the mystical Western tradition such as Meister Ekhart, William James, Richard Bucke, and F. C. Happold.

Surveys have revealed that almost 70% of persons have such a transcendent experience at some time in their lives. Our challenge is to help individuals gain the skill to capture this experience *at will* to condition their health in a positive way. Practicing regular meditation can achieve this aim (see appendix 2). Descriptions of these states of consciousness describe peace, unity, atonement, bliss, joy, and an understanding of how everything in our life is connected. The effect of these states on daily life is to enhance health and well-being, and even in cases of incurable disease an acceptance and quiet joy can be experienced. Community health centers in various parts of the world are now offering stress-reduction programs; the Mindfulness Based Stress Reduction program in Meriden, Connecticut, is an impressive example.[12]

When I use esoteric healing, my clients often start to experience the qualities just mentioned and describe the experience as total relaxation and peace, even though they also feel energized. After a few sessions, I may suggest that they can learn this technique and practice it on themselves, relatives, and friends. Frequently, in time, they become students of this healing approach. I mention this here to indicate that the esoteric healing described in this book is a skill anyone can learn. Nor do people have to go through some kind of "initiatory" experience with a teacher who passes on some kind of "power." The capacity to contact our own healing essence or soul belongs to everyone. We just need to remove the inner blockages to elicit this healing flow from the soul.

Twenty-first century life is already very busy, and this fact is the main antagonistic factor for our healing because we leave no time for the soul. I have noticed that the average client is more stressed now than ten years ago. People are working longer hours and are afraid of losing their jobs if they take time off; personal relationships are more stressed. As a result, tiredness and exhaustion are endemic. I did a health survey in my practice during the 1970s and found nervous complaints were the most common category for consultations. If a survey were to be done today I think this factor would be even more prominent. Such nervous disorders include exhaustion, tension, insomnia, poor concentration, anxiety, and low libido.

Energy Dissipation through Excessive Busyness

The chief subtle factor in disease today is probably excessive activity in too many directions. This dissipation of energy affects our thoughts and emotions, causing a jumble of thoughts and, in time, stimulating negative emotions such as depression, anger, and resentment. In my clinic, I find it necessary to remind nearly all our clients about their appointments. Sometimes they forget, even if I remind them the day before. This tendency has greatly increased over the last ten years, and other therapists tell me the same story.

There is a tremendous expectation on improving our performance today at work, at home, in sexuality, or on the sports field. This ambitious striving prevents us from living in the present and savoring life as it is in any moment. Krishnamurti was one of the great teachers of the art of living in the moment, and his *Commentaries on Living* is well worth reading for the purpose of understanding the value of becoming unconditioned from the past or future.[13] When we are truly present at any particular moment, we can more adequately act and respond to the needs of that moment. It is essential for our health to make a quiet space a couple of times each day to re-collect, center, and be in stillness so as to sense the peace and purpose flowing from our inner self (techniques for this are discussed later).

Negative Emotions As a Disease Cause

Negative emotions are a major cause of disease. Over the last fifty years, techniques for owning and exploring our emotions have featured in the practice of many psychologists and self-help groups. It is of value to reflect on how *transparent* we have become in this respect. Many individuals now share their emotions freely within the family and work life. However, I find in clinical practice there is an enormous amount of emotional blackmail still taking place in family life, between individuals, and in the workplace. In other words, individuals manipulate each other, often in very subtle ways, for their own benefit. An example would be a mother who pushes her husband to work harder so that their daughters can go to an expensive school, not because the education there is superior, but for her own self-esteem.

Tremendous pressures are put on children to achieve at school and university. Appalling scenarios take place, involving access to children in the case of divorced and separated couples; unbelievable attitudes are expressed in relation to elderly people and their wills. Even less extreme emotional dramas can cause exhaustion of the nervous system and result in clinical stress.

Apparently, the nerve toxins caused by negative emotions are amongst the most toxic that we can develop. Thanks largely to the medical research of Candice Pert, we now know that "the molecules of emotion," as her book calls them, can affect cell receptors involving the immune system in every part of our body.[14] Hence, the common saying, "I have a gut feeling" is literally true. We begin to see how closely the inner factors for disease are connected to the outer ones. In particular, our energy field, with its accompanying electromagnetic field, is profoundly conditioned by our thoughts and emotions.

The Energy Field or Etheric Body

Just as the brain is the hard wiring and computer-like interface for our emotions and thoughts, we have a more subtle structure for our consciousness, which underlies our brain and nervous system. This structure is called the energy field, or etheric body, and is the means for our soul to express itself in the outer world. The etheric body is the bridge between our higher states of consciousness and the physical brain. It has always seemed logical to me that we would have a pathway for our subtle consciousness rather than just having a soul floating around like a captive balloon attached to our body by unknown means.

The discoveries of physicists in the twentieth century have made it easier to bridge science and religion, although many of the attempts seem clumsy compared to the detailed treatises from Eastern philosophers. Science now describes space as related to the concept of the quantum vacuum, which is understood to be a very high state of energy providing enormous pressure per square inch. So rather than containing nothing, space is thought to contain the energy from which our tangible universe develops.

This makes it easier to understand that the physical body may have subtle mechanisms underlying it that we cannot discern with our five senses. There are a number of descriptions by different authors who basically agree about the structure of our subtle anatomy or etheric body. I will briefly describe some of its key features so that the inner causes of disease may be clearer.

The etheric body can be considered as the blueprint for the development and growth of the physical body. It is composed of subtle matter that, in one sense, is still physical but is more subtle than solids, liquids, and gases, and, therefore, unable to be measured by the current instruments of physics. However, its mirror image, our electromagnetic field, can be measured by electronic instruments and therefore, indirectly, we can have a scientific evaluation of the etheric state. Professor William Tiller uses the term "magneto-electric" for the etheric body, and he sees the electromagnetic field as a mirror image of the etheric.[15] Researchers Harold Saxton Burr, Valerie Hunt, and Harry Oldfield have used electronic equipment to indirectly measure the etheric field in this way.[16]

The etheric body interpenetrates and extends beyond the physical body. It is seen by many people with extrasensory perception as a shimmering golden network or, at times, as bluish-white. Within our etheric field are areas of great activity or vortices of force that are traditionally known as the chakras, which is from the Sanskrit and means "wheels." The energies of the etheric are concentrated in the areas of the chakras, and the weaving of the energies gives the appearance of petals. There are seven major chakras or energy centers aligned vertically from the base of the spine to the top of the head, and the energies become more complex the higher we move up the spine. The base chakra appears to have four petals while the head centers have many hundreds of petals.

Each of the seven major chakras relates to a different state of consciousness, while the chakras above the diaphragm relate to higher states of consciousness, which is why they are more complex. In addition to the major chakras, there are 21 minor chakras associated with individual organs such as the eyes, ears, kidneys, and ovaries. Others are situated in the palms of the hands, behind the knees, on the soles of the feet, and a further 49 focal points, scattered throughout the body. Still smaller centers relate to the hundreds of acupuncture points of the Chinese meridian system, which is also part of the etheric body.

Since the 1990s, some prominent medical and physical scientists have written extensively on how to validate the chakra system from a scientific viewpoint. One such person is the aforementioned William Tiller, professor of material sciences in the engineering department at Stanford University in Palo Alto, California. He views the chakras as electrical transformers that step down or step up the body energies. His research includes a thorough study of Eastern concepts such as the chakra system, nadis (minor energy lines in the body), and the meridians. He regards the chakra system as related to the nadis of the Hindu system and has described them as antennae that receive physical and subtle signals from the environment of the person. These signals are then transduced by electrical means to be received by the nervous system and endocrine glands.

Tiller says: "The chakra/endocrine gland/neural plexus system transfers subtle energies of various types to our bodies via a power stepdown and field transduction process. These energies fuel the hormonal factories of the glands and vitalize the central nervous system. Analogous processes occur at the etheric level and these interact closely with the acupuncture meridian system."[17]

The seven major chakras or centers can therefore be considered as electrical transformers stepping the energy down from our emotions, thoughts, and higher states of consciousness so as to be comfortably received by our nervous system and all parts of our physical body. Thus our states of consciousness, thoughts, and emotions have a profound effect on the chakras and the etheric body. For example, if an individual is very angry his solar plexus chakra will become distorted and there may be an excessive flow of energy via the chakra to the stomach, resulting in severe indigestion. The etheric can be considered as the mediator of our inner states to the physical body. Our immunity to disease is conditioned by the state of our etheric field and its accompanying electromagnetic field.

In its role as mediator, the etheric body can also be affected from the outside by man-made electromagnetic interference and by certain chemicals. Hallucinogenic drugs such as morphine, heroin, and marijuana have a profound and detrimental effect on the etheric body. It is therefore subject to assaults from both inner and outer factors, indicating again the subtle relationship between these two aspects of disease.

The Functions of the Etheric Body

The etheric body has several important functions:

1) To act as a blueprint or pattern for all the cells and tissues of the body in terms of growth and for healing following disease or injury.

2) To act as the mediator between higher states of consciousness and the brain via the seven major chakras.

3) To transmit energy to all parts of the body.

The etheric body is intimately related to our level of energy and our vitality. It can be tight and finely woven like a piece of silk, or, at the opposite end of the vitality scale, it can be like an unstrung tennis racquet. The etheric body not only interpenetrates the physical body, but also radiates outwards and is called the health aura. As mentioned, it is not possible to measure the etheric body directly with instruments of science, but its associated electromagnetic field is amenable to measurement. The term bio-magnetism is often used to describe the electromagnetic field surrounding the body.

Until recently, the etheric body has been difficult to define or measure in relation to health and disease. We all know how it feels to have plenty of energy, but how do we measure this? If medical scientists are skeptical about what natural therapists mean by toxins, they have been even more critical of the concept of vitalism that has featured so strongly in naturopathic medicine for 200 years. But science has established through the super quantum interference device (SQUID) that living bodies are surrounded by oscillating or vibrating magnetic fields. It is through these fields that healers can affect the energy field and etheric body of another individual. As reported by James Oschman in *Energy Medicine*, energy effects from a healer have been measured by SQUIDs; all healing approaches such as Reiki, pranic healing, Therapeutic Touch, or Healing Touch, produce similar effects in terms of magnetic fields.[18]

In addition, medical scientist Robert Becker has established that we have a magnetic sense involving crystals of magnetite situated deep within the brain near the pineal gland. Therefore, we can also sense and diagnose the magnetic field of another person by focusing on the condition of their magnetic field. I was taught this process by Fran Nixon, a Canadian woman, in 1980; she called this technique of energy diagnosis "finding the ion flow," and I have used the faculty in my naturopathic practice ever since. My previous book, *The Vivaxis Connection*, details these easily learned techniques.[19] Over the years, I have reinterpreted the findings of Fran Nixon for my medical work.

There is some scientific basis for this term, because in all cases of illness the ion flow is found to indicate a disturbance of energies. So, later in this book, when I mention doing an "energy scan" on a client, you will know that I am referring to the technique of establishing whether there is a healthy energy flow in the organs.

Shortly after learning the Vivaxis technique, I realized that it was connected to the heartbeat, and I now view this energy flow as related to the magnetic field of the heart. Two American researchers, Gary Schwartz and Linda Russek, have written pioneering papers on the use of the heart to diagnose all kinds of illness. In traditional Chinese medicine, the pulse diagnosis is very basic to this system. Schwartz and Russek have taken this system of diagnosis into the twenty-first century by indicating how modern medical science can use the heartbeat for the purpose of diagnosis.[20]

In my naturopathic practice, I use the human magnetic sense to diagnose the health of the energy field, chakras, and organs. This simple technique can be learned by 90% of individuals in a few days. It is simply a slight variation of the skill needed to use a pendulum or dowsing rod.

A cardiologist named Irving Dardik, M.D., has written a revealing paper on the relationship between the rhythm of the heartbeat and all types of chronic disease. He has demonstrated that heart rate variability lessens in such disease. In other words, if we are healthy, there are minute variations in the intervals between heartbeats, whereas in all chronic disease there is an entrenched rhythm that does not allow for adaptation to changing needs of the body. Like the previously mentioned researchers, Dr. Dardik has illustrated his findings via magnetic resonance rather than relying on the electrical pattern as illustrated by the electrocardiograph. The magnetic picture gives much more detail of heart function.[21] (See part 2 in the chapter on heart and circulatory problems.)

Diagnosing the Inner Cause of Disease

In my naturopathic practice, I use the human magnetic sense to diagnose the health of the energy field, chakras, and organs. This simple technique can be learned by 90% of individuals in a few days. It

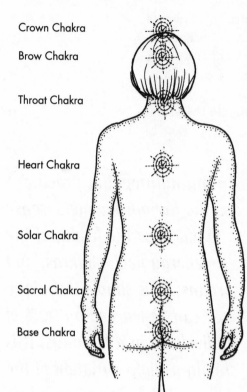

Crown Chakra	Pineal gland, upper brain, right eye. Reception of spiritual light and impressions. Synthesis of all energies.
Brow Chakra	Pituitary gland, lower brain, left eye, ears, and sinuses. Spiritual or personality, ambition. Distributor of spiritual energies.
Throat Chakra	Thyroid gland, upper respiratory system, lymphatic system. Mental creativity, planning and scheming. Manipulation of energy.
Heart Chakra	Thymus gland, circulatory system, lungs, and breasts. Love/wisdom. Empathy and understanding. Inclusiveness.
Solar Chakra	Pancreas, digestive system. Sympathy. Desires. Aspirations. Emotional identification.
Sacral Chakra	Reproductive system, ovaries and testes. Pleasures, comforts. Wise use of food and sex. Positive use of money.
Base Chakra	Adrenals, kidneys, and spine. Will to live, Basic energy. Grounding.

FIGURE 2: THE SEVEN CHAKRAS AND ASSOCIATED QUALITIES. Illustrates input of chakras in relation to the spine and the head.

is simply a slight variation of the skill needed to use a pendulum or dowsing rod. I have found that not only the human energy field, but also all living things on our planet, including plants and animals, have a basic pulsation. In the case of the vegetable kingdom, this probably relates to the flow of water or sap through the plant material. In the healthy state, everything on our planet is conditioned by the natural and healthy magnetic field of the Earth, and this magnetic field oscillates from 7–10 cycles per second. So important to health is this field that NASA now simulates this frequency in the space capsules where the astronauts work and live so as to preserve their health.

When there is a disturbance caused by blocked or short-circuited energy, a chaotic energy pattern ensues. The cause can be chemical or electromagnetic. If the body becomes diseased or injured, subtle healing can help restore the etheric body and its associated magnetic field to its normal state, and the healing of the physical organs and tissues is hastened thereby. You will realize from a consideration of the functions in relation to the etheric body how important it is to keep it in good health and to prevent disturbance from chemical and electromagnetic sources. Other subtler energy fields associated with different levels of consciousness surround and interpenetrate the etheric field and thus condition it further.

The Chain of Inner Causes

The etheric body is conditioned by whatever is our habitual mode of being. For instance, we may be a very emotionally expressive person, constantly swinging between hilarity and depression—almost bipolar. Or we may get angry, jealous, or resentful very easily. The etheric will be conditioned by these emotions, and this will, in turn, affect the physical organs via the chakras and meridian system.

For example, I have found that a number of hemorrhoid sufferers carry resentment. People with gallstones frequently suppress anger and irritation and may even harbor hatred in their psyche. I have noticed that cancer below the diaphragm appears more common in persons who suppress their emotional life, and breast cancer has been associated in many of my clients with an old and deep grief. However, in cancer, and indeed, in most illness, there will usually be other associated outer causes, such as deficiencies of antioxidants, minerals, and vitamins, plus inherited tendencies.

Other people are conditioned more from the mental level rather than the emotional. This does not mean that they necessarily suppress their emotions, but they may be more interested in study, accumulating knowledge, and in general developing their minds. I have noticed that an aberration of the mentally alert person can manifest as a tendency for crystallized thoughts in some direction—for instance, excessive thoughts about health. Often, in the iris of such persons, I will see signs of crystallization in the physical body. This may manifest as hardened arteries or stones in the kidneys or gallbladder. Again, there may be corresponding outer causes, such as a lack of magnesium, causing their calcium to be out of balance. "Acid" thoughts may also result in accumulation of uric acid in organs and tissues.

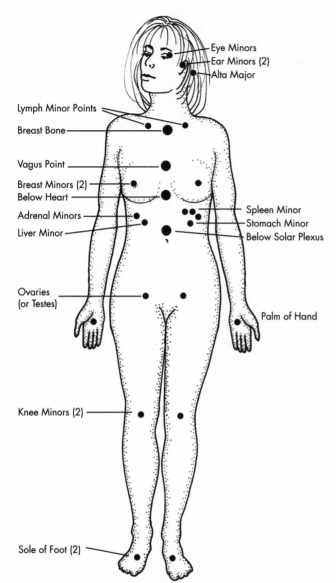

Eye Minors
Ear Minors (2)
Alta Major

Lymph Minor Points

Breast Bone

Vagus Point

Breast Minors (2)
Below Heart

Adrenal Minors

Liver Minor

Spleen Minor
Stomach Minor
Below Solar Plexus

Ovaries
(or Testes)

Palm of Hand

Knee Minors (2)

Sole of Foot (2)

FIGURE 3: MINOR CHAKRAS.

It is the chakras or energy centers that transmit thoughts and emotions into the etheric body. They are the mechanism for the transmission of energy, and they step it down from one level to another. The chakras therefore have counterparts at the mental, emotional, and etheric levels and are the transmitters of energy from those spheres of energy. Figure 2 depicts the major qualities associated with each chakra, while figure 3 shows the minor chakras.

I find that most of my clients have heard about the chakras, but very few understand the mechanisms of our subtle constitution. It has always surprised me that psychologists are not interested in searching more widely for a mechanism that might express our thoughts and feelings. Among psychologists and medical scientists, there appears to be a prevailing concept that thoughts and emotions are somehow an offshoot of the brain.

However, evidence from near-death and out-of-the-body experiences has interested some scientists in undertaking serious thought as to new explanations for the mechanisms of consciousness. A few psychologists and psychiatrists now postulate that our mental and emotional consciousness can be independent from the body. In the future, psychologists may become just as interested in the mechanism for consciousness involving the chakra system as they have hitherto been in examining the brain and nervous system and the five physical senses.

The twentieth-century physicist Albert Einstein enabled us to understand more easily how energy is related to mass. We now know that the solid objects in our environment are dense manifestations of energy, and it is logical to make a case for our own physical body being associated with fields of energy. Writers with scientific backgrounds have attempted to fit the Eastern concept of the universe and the human constitution to the findings of twentieth-century physics. The main problem here seems to be one of oversimplification.

For instance, having explained that there is a "sea" of virtual energy underlying our physical universe, some scientists talk about the possibility of the physical universe and also our consciousness as being waves on the surface of this "quantum sea." Our immortality after physical death is therefore understood to be a small wave, merging again with the quantum sea. This scenario is not comforting to the average intelligent person who looks for continuity of consciousness following their many life endeavors.

Indeed, there are lots of gaps in quantum theory, and thinkers in the East and West have developed the concept of a more hierarchical universe. The virtual energy in the quantum vacuum mentioned by physicists is probably only one of many interpenetrating fields beyond. So we should not equate the quantum vacuum with the ultimate level of being. Rather than losing our individual awareness by merging into the quantum sea after death, it may be, according to surveys of near death and other spiritual experiences, that after death, we continue to exist in other spheres until our consciousness finally, after many further lives, becomes omniscient or all-embracing. At this stage some merging with an ultimate level of being would seem appropriate.

So my model for the inner causes of disease is hierarchical. I know that some people have a problem with hierarchies, but hierarchy is a fact in our environment. For instance, we know that there are electrons within atoms within molecules within cells within tissues within organs. That's a hierarchy. So why not hierarchy in terms of our personal consciousness? The model I present views the human constitution as being composed of many energy fields that interpenetrate one another and are composed of increasingly subtle energy as we move through the etheric, astral, mental, and soul levels

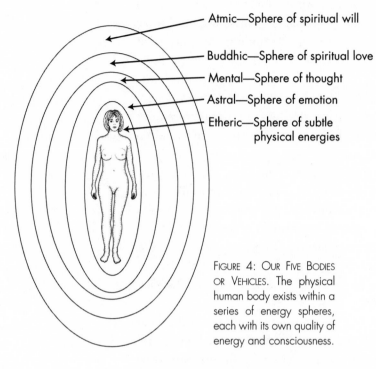

Atmic—Sphere of spiritual will

Buddhic—Sphere of spiritual love

Mental—Sphere of thought

Astral—Sphere of emotion

Etheric—Sphere of subtle
physical energies

FIGURE 4: OUR FIVE BODIES
OR VEHICLES. The physical
human body exists within a
series of energy spheres,
each with its own quality of
energy and consciousness.

(see figure 4). After all, today "increasingly subtle energy" implies a hierarchy.

The Subtle Fields of Consciousness

One way to envisage our mechanism for consciousness is to picture those Russian dolls, in which there is a doll within a doll within a doll. Another analogy is to imagine the various ever-finer substances of our consciousness as interpenetrating, like air within water within earth. I like this analogy better than the Russian dolls because these various substances are not in separate spaces as with the dolls. It is also appropriate because metaphysicians often equate the physical body with the elements of earth, the emotions with water, and the mind with air or fire.

In this chapter, I have presented the model of the human as one that is self-evident if we reflect on our experience of life and being. Extending the above concepts, our personality can be thought to consist of a physical/etheric body that has sensations such as temperature, pleasure, pain, etc.; of a further body or energy field that is composed of emotions, desires, and feelings; and of another body that contains and creates our thoughts. Then we have three more subtle levels of functioning related to our creative intelligence, capacity for universal love, and for spiritual will.

We can say that the lower three bodies comprise our personality and are a reflection in time and space of the higher three. It is the higher levels of consciousness that seem to be activated in the transcendent experiences mentioned earlier. Mediating between these higher and lower functions is the soul—our central principle.

As electrical transformers, the chakras step down the energy of the various fields of consciousness so that our brain and nervous system can respond without being blown apart by the energies contacted. We have a chakra that corresponds with each level of consciousness, and, in addition, each chakra corresponds to an endocrine gland and its associated organs. So in the case of the solar plexus, for instance, there is a flow of energy from our astral or body of emotions via its gateway, the solar plexus chakra, into the associated gland, the pancreas, and from thence to all the digestive organs.

In the case of digestive problems, there may be particular emotions, such as anger or depression, that cause a contraction in the solar plexus chakra that, in turn, inhibits the flow of hormones from the pancreas and the flow of digestive juices. The end result may be an inability to digest certain foodstuffs, giving rise to food sensitivities and, in extreme cases, to allergies. There may be accompanying diarrhea or constipation and abdominal pains, due to spasm of the small and/or large bowel. This is often called irritable bowel syndrome, and, if combined with poor diet, it causes an accumulation of toxins that may eventually develop into ulcerative colitis or bowel cancer.

You can see how the natural therapist does not see a condition in isolation from the rest of the body functions as often happens in orthodox medicine. In the scenario mentioned above, the inner psychic manifestations of particular emotions are also included. The role of the healer is to shift the focus of the client from the physical problem to the soul. This can be achieved in different ways as, for instance, with meditation or healing. However, before detailing this healing process, I want to describe the possible healing path. This path involves the invoking of energy from our soul to move through the chakra system in particular stages; these can be seen as three basic transmutations from the lower to the higher chakras. With this in mind, the healing process can be better understood.

The American psychologist Abraham Maslow demonstrated in the twentieth century the hierarchy of needs in terms of consciousness. He found that a person tends to shift their focus from physical to emotional to mental to spiritual concerns.[22] His research showed that people experience transcendent experiences more often when their basic needs for physical comfort and emotional security are satisfied. Of course, we can think of examples where spiritual striving has taken place *due* to severe deprivations that provoked spiritual experiences, but these are rare cases.

It seems logical to me that we can associate subtle fields with our various states of consciousness whose subtlety increases as we move from physical sensations to transcendent or spiritual levels. Even the soul can be considered as having a "body," even if of the finest sub-stance. In fact, the soul could be considered as the center point between the worlds of form and transcendence. The soul is often called the middle principle, mediating between spirit and matter. Returning to the opening thoughts of this chapter, we should aim to have the soul address and condition our etheric body, for it is then that perfect health results.

Our train of energy transmission on the inside should start with the soul. It is for this reason that the esoteric healer aligns with her own soul with the aim of invoking the healing from the soul of the client in the healing process. We will explore this in the next chap-ter. The inner chain of conditioning causes responsible for health or disease goes like this: *our soul body → mental body/mental chakras → astral body/astral chakras → etheric body/etheric chakras → physical body and organs.*

The Health Consequences of Stagnant Thought-Forms

When considering the inner factors of thought and emotions, our main need for health is to have a free flow of energy through the mind (or mental body), the astral body (understood as another subtle sheath related to our emotions), and etheric body. Most people understand that blockages cause health problems, and people talk of having an emotional or mental block. It is hard to go through life without becoming conditioned in certain directions, and this causes a slowing down or stasis of energy. Remember the earlier reference to the busyness of twenty-first-century living and its consequent dissi-pation of energy in all directions.

We therefore often find a twofold problem at the inner level. First, there is a whirling of unfocused energies in all directions, resulting in exhaustion and frustration due to lack of achievement of particular goals. Second, areas in the psyche with stagnant thought-forms become barriers to the flow of healthy energies. The general busyness of the person may often prevent adequate attention being given to the blockages. In many cases, there is some awareness of crystallization and conditioning, but the person may deliberately keep busy so as to have an excuse not to attend to the areas that need attention.

In some cases, especially those of child sexual abuse, I have noted persistent thought-forms associated with the sacral chakra, and I have used techniques to remove them. We all suffer from some fixations at the emotional or mental level, and in many cases these are caused by our cultural conditioning; they will particularly affect the lower chakras. Caroline Myss is well-known for her work and writing in this area of "tribal roots" and cultural connections in relation to the chakras. She especially focuses on the three chakras below the diaphragm, and indeed it is these chakras that correspond to those levels of our consciousness that are conditioned by family, race, culture, and religion.[23]

Summary: The main focus in healing should be to align to our inner essence or soul so that healing energy can flow through to the physical body. The mediator between our soul consciousness, psyche, and brain consciousness is the etheric body, which has a number of important functions for physical health. Our physical body is inter-penetrated by this etheric body. In addition, our psyche consists of a number of energy fields within which are found transforming and transmitting centers known as chakras. These energy fields correspond to our feeling nature, mind, and higher states of consciousness, the accessing of which is often called a transcendent experience. Our energy fields and psyche condition our etheric body and therefore affect our health.

The chakras are related to the Chinese meridian system, and we therefore have a hierarchy or chain, which connects our soul with mind, emotions, etheric body, chakras, meridian system, nervous system, blood circulation, organs, and tissues. Disease results from an interruption of energy at *any* level in this chain. The therapist can learn simple techniques to evaluate the energy field around the body without the use of instruments.

Modern physics has given us clues about the universe that indicate the possibility of understanding how energy fields may underlie the human physical body. A number of medical researchers are starting to provide a framework to understand the chakra system and the effect of our psyche on our health. Science has also provided an instrument known by the acronym SQUID to measure the magnetic energy field around the body; the healing effect from the healer can also be measured by this instrument.

4 The Chakras—
Mechanisms for
Soul Expression

In this chapter, I explore the chakras in a different way from other writings on the subject (including my own previous books) by placing more emphasis on their *connection* to our daily life. The terms "chakras" and "energy centers" will be used interchangeably. The three chakras at and below the diaphragm relate to the personal life as lived by the average person. Here, there will be a strong expression of national and cultural roots, plus a life often governed by a sense of family ties. Making sufficient money for a comfortable life in terms of home, car, clothes, food, holidays, and entertainment features strongly here. There could be an emphasis on sporting interests with passionate loyalties to the home side. All of these personal expressions relate to the lower three chakras—the base, sacral, and solar plexus.

The four chakras above the diaphragm relate to developments in our life that have a more universal application. In other words, the higher chakras develop when we take the focus off our personal interests and become more concerned with serving humanity and the planet in any creative avenue. This service may not be of the type normally considered as spiritual and may have nothing to do with churches, meditation, or the mystical life. It could be in the area of politics, health and medicine, education, the arts, science, or finance.

We need to think of "spiritual" as a process that enlarges our understanding by achieving creative growth in some area. To develop spiritually is to grow in a sense that is positive for self, others, and/or the environment. It has nothing to do with going to church or following a spiritual leader. One of the most significant of Christ's sayings in the New Testament is, "By their fruits will ye know them."

In terms of our health, the differences in expression between the lower and higher chakras will have a profound effect. Any life function that is over-emphasized will be likely to cause a congestion or blockage of energy that will prevent energies flowing freely through all the chakras.

> *For instance, if a person is obsessed with making money, then we could expect a blockage or over-activity in the sacral chakra, the center related to our ability to earn money. If a mother is obsessed with the welfare of her child and tries to keep even an adult child "tied to her apron strings," there will be an over-activity of the solar plexus chakra.*

For instance, if a person is obsessed with making money, then we could expect a blockage or over-activity in the sacral chakra, the center related to our ability to earn money. If a mother is obsessed with the welfare of her child and tries to keep even an adult child "tied to her apron strings," there will be an over-activity of the solar plexus chakra. This chakra is involved with conditional love and affection, as distinct from the unconditional love of the heart. Chakra disturbances will affect the related organs and tissues.

Each chakra below the diaphragm relates to one above it. As we grow on life's journey, the energies from the lower chakras are transmuted into energies with more universal application via the higher chakras. It is most useful to study the chakras as three pairs because there are three basic transmutations: from physical to mental creativity (sacral→throat); selfish and personal love to universal love (solar plexus→heart); and personal will to spiritual will (base→crown).

The brow chakra can be considered as an extension of the sacral/throat pair because it is concerned with ideas. Energies flow both ways through the brow chakra. Initially, it synthesizes all the energies of the spinal chakras representing the personality life; then it receives energies from the soul via the crown chakra and distributes these energies, for instance, in healing.

Each chakra should be considered as a sphere that connects with the major nerve plexi on either side of the spine. For practical purposes, we can consider that they have inlets behind the spine and outlets in the front of the body. When we are healthy and balanced, the chakras are roughly equal in size to each other, and there should be an equal flow of energy from the back and front of each chakra.

The energy seems to flow into the main chakras from each level of consciousness on the spinal side. However, as the chakras act like vortexes, this movement through the spine is difficult to describe. The energies spin through the chakras and pass to the associated glands and organs. The size of the chakras, if measured from side to side, depends on the strength of the energies as they spin and flow through each chakra. Thus, if any chakra is temporarily depleted of energy, its size or circumference will be smaller. Furthermore, when comparing one person with another the size of the chakras will vary considerably, depending on the emotional, mental, and spiritual development of the persons involved.

Because each chakra transmits different energies from our fields of awareness—for instance, physical, emotional, mental, or spiritual, according to our changing focus—the chakras will vary in size from time to time. They therefore tend to get out of balance if there is too much focus on one level of consciousness, and this is eventually reflected in the physical glands. If, for instance, the throat chakra is bigger than the others, it indicates an excess of energy in that area, which can disturb the associated thyroid gland and throat tissues.

Ideally, each of our chakras should be the same size. After we do the esoteric healing, any imbalance in size is corrected. It will depend on the lifestyle and psychology of the person involved as to whether this balance is maintained.

Although the base center is the first chakra, counting upwards, we will start our journey with the sacral/throat pair, as they express the first energies that manifest strongly in our development. After the three pairs are considered, we will look at the remaining two head centers and the spleen. You will see that the associated gland and its health or disease always gives us a clue to the functioning and energies of the related chakra.

The Sacral Chakra: Food, Sex, and Comforts

The sacral center is located at the level of the lower back known as the sacroiliac joint and in the front just above the pubic bone. The glands associated with the sacral center are the gonads—the ovaries in the female and testes in the male. The associated tissues are connected with the reproductive system including ovaries, fallopian tubes, uterus, and vagina in the female, and testes and prostate in the male. The lower part of the large bowel is also associated with this chakra.

Disturbance of this energy center will, therefore, involve any of these tissues and could include cystic ovaries, uterine fibroids, menstrual irregularities, infertility in both sexes, prostatitis, cancer in any part of the reproductive system, and lower bowel problems such as constipation. At the psychological level, sexual problems may manifest. The sacral chakra expresses our ability to handle prana and etheric energy in general. This manifests as interest in food, sex, and comfort. Our intimate relationships will be conditioned by the health of this chakra. Promiscuity can obviously result in sexually transmitted disease such as venereal herpes and warts, gonorrhea, syphilis, chlamydia, and AIDS.

All these conditions can result from over-activity of this chakra. Generally speaking, the sacral center is connected with creativity, in terms of sexual relationships and the perpetuation of the species. If we reflect on the focus of television advertisements and programs, we note that 99% feature overt or subtle references to food, sex, or comforts in our living space. Hence, there is an enormous focus within humanity on the functions of the chakras below the diaphragm. Our intimate relationships, family connections, and basic desires for pleasure and entertainment express strongly through the sacral chakra. If we think of the development of the small child or even our domestic animals, we can see an emphasis on the will to survive (base center) and need for food, comfort, and close physical contact (sacral center).

As we consider each chakra, we can understand its activity from reflecting on the connections and function of its associated gland. The associated endocrine glands here are the ovaries and testes. As with the adrenal glands, there are far-reaching connections throughout the body involving the gonads. If the levels of estrogen and progesterone drop too suddenly in women of any age, there can be depression, low libido, insomnia, exhaustion, and poor concentration.

It is of significance that modern life is so hectic that many of my female clients complain of exhaustion and low libido long before the age of menopause. From my viewpoint, this happens when the base chakra and adrenals start to become exhausted; then the sacral center and ovaries start to slow down. This illustrates the connections between the centers and the glands. Interestingly, women are less likely to compartmentalize their energies than men. Perhaps due to the instinct to survive or for family reasons, their libido is the first energy to often completely disappear when their health is threatened. Men, on the other hand, are often known to continue with high levels of libido when other aspects of their health are threatened.

Sacral Chakra Case History: Loretta is a nun who does a small amount of remedial teaching in her retirement. She suffered from an autoimmune disease called lupus, and this syndrome often affects the joints, kidneys, skin, and even the brain. This is an inherited predisposition from the medical and naturopathic viewpoints. Loretta also had Raynaud's Syndrome, which can often go with lupus; this syndrome affects the circulation of the hands. She also suffered bad headaches and constipation.

The main reason for including this case history here is to show the effect of the mind on the chakras. Loretta always felt better after having a healing. However, I was interested to find when I scanned her chakras that the sacral center was imbalanced at the mental level; it was much larger than the other chakras at that level of consciousness. Later when reflecting on this anomaly, I realized that, as a nun, she may not have had any normal sexual experience and thus her mind was perhaps curious and dwelling on sexual matters. I wondered what effect this might have on her immune system.

It was significant that Loretta had undergone a total hysterectomy for fibroids earlier in her life, indicating, perhaps, a long-standing problem with the sacral chakra. However, there are cases where you realize that a discussion on such matters is not appropriate. Her chronic disease was well advanced and she did not appear to have the temperament for any vital change at the psychological level.

At the physical level, she did quite well on vitamin C for general detoxifying, magnesium orotate for the spasm in her hands, and a mixture of herbs for her immune system and liver. She also took an organic iron tablet for anemia, and a herbal tablet for arthritis in her spine. Liver and lymphatic cleansing homeopathics were combined with a deep-acting miasmatic remedy called Thuja for her inherited predispositions. As a result of these treatments, Loretta had improvements with her constipation, circulation, and headaches.

The Throat Chakra: Our Creativity

The higher counterpart of the sacral is the throat center, situated around the base of the neck at the seventh cervical vertebra, the one that feels like a big knob. The associated endocrine gland is the thyroid, located in front of the voice box or larynx. This gland controls the rate of our metabolism, and if it is overactive we have a condition called hyperthyroidism or toxic goiter. In this disorder, body processes are speeded up and we have fast heartbeat, possibly high blood pressure, weight loss, and increased peristalsis or bowel movements. Anxiety, sweating, and nervousness can also be featured. Due to the speed of modern living, this condition is becoming more common and is due to too much energy flowing through the throat chakra or to an inability to fully use such energy.

The opposite condition is also common and is called hypothyroidism or simple goiter. This can occur from a lack of iodine in the diet, but it also occurs when there is not enough creative activity in the life of the person concerned. I have had numerous cases in which I have perceived a deficiency in the throat chakra and the client has admitted being disturbed or frustrated by having no real creativity in their life. This does not mean that they are not busy; we can be very busy without experiencing the joy of creativity.

The throat chakra becomes vitalized when we start to make a creative contribution to life. It then draws up the energy from the sacral center and a balance starts to take place between the two. The energy of the sacral center is needed to attract the needed money and labor for the creative schemes of the throat chakra. We all know people who are always scheming, but their schemes come to naught because they do not have the right balance between the sacral center and the throat.

The development of radio, television, satellite communication, the computer, and now the Internet have manifested as a result of throat chakra energy within humanity. These developments are all to do with communication and the voice of humanity. By reflecting on the content of Internet material, we realize that a lot of material is an expression of the sacral center—shopping, entertainment, pornography—while other material is educational, inspiring, and spiritually motivated. The Internet is a perfect example of sacral/throat interaction and illustrates how the chakras can externalize their energies within humanity as a whole.

Due to the changes at menopause when the ovaries shut down, the shift of energies in a woman is more noticeable than in the male. Menopause is the time when the children, if she has any, are off her hands, and she often begins to live for herself, perhaps for the first time. Ideally, women should develop some creative activity *before* menopause so that they can increase the output of creative work as a result of more time and energy after children leave the nest and after menopause.

Due to the creative shift within the whole of humanity, we find that the level of creativity has already reached an all-time high, even in young people. Economic changes and technology have provided the opportunity for the most amazing array of ingenious activity. The emphasis is off childbearing for many couples, and this may be a reason for the increase of infertility observed in both sexes. I find in my practice that many persons are also querying the cycles in their lives when sex is no longer of much interest. It is helpful to explain the shift from the sacral to the throat that is taking place on a large scale within the leading edge of human consciousness, because the expectation to perform adequately in the sexual area has increased over the last thirty years.

Hence, in any intimate partnership, one person may lose interest in sex to some extent because their energies are focused increasingly through the throat center in some artistic pursuit. At the same time, their self-esteem plunges, because the other partner expects a better sexual performance due to being more focused in consciousness through the sacral center. An understanding of the associations with each chakra may thus help our relationships.

So what are the implications of the sacral/throat axis for our health? We need to learn to eliminate the nonessentials from our life so that there is space to be creative without too much pressure. Over busyness is likely to lead to an over-active throat chakra. Lack of effort to develop creative outlets is likely to result in an under-active throat chakra and to depression, which is being described as the disease of the twenty-first century. If you remember those times when you are creative, you will note that depression rarely occurs. Frustration of our creative needs and the associated lack of self-esteem is a major cause of depression and are related to frustration of our ideals in life.

I have noticed that osteoarthritis of the fingers in women over fifty can be related to a lack of creative outlet in their life. The choice of creativity can range from gardening, painting, sewing, writing, singing, and running a successful business, to creative living in the home. People seem to be most satisfied when their creative activity is appreciated and used by others. The outflow from the throat chakra then becomes of a more universal nature.

Other health problems from the imbalance of the throat chakra relate to the associated tissues of the larynx, throat, bronchial tree, upper lungs, and lymphatic system. Disorders will therefore include laryngitis, bronchitis, asthma, and mucous discharges from the throat and bronchials. It is in these conditions that we see a combination of the inner and outer causes of disease.

Outer factors include the many airborne pollutants plus poor diet, which can lead to an accumulation of toxins in the lymphatic system and breathing apparatus. Inherited factors will also add to the disease tendency for bronchial troubles or osteoarthritis. It is interesting that in asthma the problem is in part an inability to breathe adequately, and this leads to very labored breathing, which leads to hyperventilation. Fear in the asthmatic often seems to be the basis for this tension that prevents the proper breathing rhythm; it may account for the success of the Buteyko Method, where clients are taught to breathe less often and less deeply. In this method, the aim is to get the body to absorb and process more carbon dioxide and thus to restrict the oxygen intake.[24]

In the twenty-first century, we have to consider the problems of the throat center and the associated bronchial tree as quite complex, due to the mixture of environmental, inherited, lifestyle, and esoteric factors. When there is an adequate flow of energies between the sacral and throat centers, the energies on their way to the throat pass through the heart, and creative activities then become also a service in some way to humanity or the planet.

Throat Chakra Case History: Joyce visited my clinic for an under-active thyroid that had been diagnosed by blood tests. She also suffered sinusitis. (Remember that the throat chakra "rules" the lymphatic system, which is usually somewhat congested in cases of chronic sinus problems.) Joyce is middle-aged and leads an active life, and she has a reasonably balanced lifestyle. I found with my technique of etheric scanning (described later) that the throat chakra was underactive, in keeping with her thyroid condition. At her first visit, Joyce was given lymphatic drainage drops combined with homeopathic kelp and another ingredient to balance the thyroid. Other remedies included vitamin B complex and the tissue salts potassium and magnesium phosphate for the nervous system.

I also included esoteric healing for Joyce and, after balancing all the chakras, I visualized triangles in her energy field relating to the flow of energy through her throat chakra (for techniques for balancing the chakras and visualizing triangles, see part 2). On her return visit, Joyce was marginally improved but the throat chakra was still a problem. We had a discussion about creativity in her life and she admitted that, although her life was very busy, she was not doing anything in which she felt creative; she wished to get back to writing.

I explained to her the connection between creativity, the throat chakra, and the thyroid gland. I also gave her a visualization whereby, after a brief meditation, she visualized or imagined triangles between her throat chakra and shoulder, then throat chakra and elbows, and finally between her throat chakra and hands. This visualization is to bring out the creative energy via her throat chakra into the environment. I generally find that clients easily imagine, for instance, lines of light connecting one chakra or part of the body to another.

Joyce only came for one more visit before moving down the coast and away from Melbourne. At that last visit, she was planning how to resume her writing career. She telephoned a month later to say that her thyroid blood test was normal even before she had actually started writing. It seems that her visualization and the planning of writing work was enough to trigger positive changes. During this period, she had no orthodox medical treatment.

The Solar Plexus Chakra: Emotions, Feelings, and Desires

Some writers on the chakras talk about the solar plexus as the seat of personal power. If we consider that all our emotions are our main source of power then I would agree, but I experience the solar plexus, in a broader sense, as transmitting all emotions. The solar plexus chakra is located in the area of the mid-dorsal vertebra when viewed from the back, and between the bottom of the sternum and the navel in the front. Think of where you feel sensations when shocked, grieving, or scared; most people will touch just above their navel. It does seem to be the focus in our body for our emotional life, and strong feelings are often registered in this area. My very young patients with night terrors often experience pain in this area.

Our emotions and feelings are related to the astral plane (which we might liken to the dream world) and to our astral or feeling body, which expresses feelings and emotions. This level of consciousness is then expressed via the solar plexus and nervous system. Of course, not only negative emotions and feelings feature through this chakra, but also feelings of happiness, loyalty, and devotion. Indeed, the full gamut of emotions and desires can be considered, ranging from the most ruthless and potentially harmful to the sublime devotion of the saint to the desire for a spiritual experience.

The concept of the solar plexus as the seat of power is best expressed in the type of emotional control that a person or persons may have over another. This may include ties between mother and child based on normal concern for the child's protection; the obsessive clinging of the devotee to the object of one's devotion; the emotional control of the dictator over his subjects; any form of emotional blackmail between persons. These could be called examples of the expression of personal power.

Power, in the sense of will, relates to the base center. However, as suggested, we cannot separate each of the lower chakras completely from each other, and there is an overlap between their functions. Thus, if a person desires to have sex with another, there will be the sensual and erotic attributes of the sacral center, the imagination and desire from the solar plexus, and the force, and possibly coercion or willfulness, from the base center. These will be intermingled in varying amounts, according to the focus of the individual and the relationship.

The pancreas is the endocrine gland associated with the solar plexus and it has both an endocrine or hormonal secretion involving insulin, and an exocrine secretion—the pancreatic juice, containing enzymes to digest carbohydrates, fats, and proteins. It is no wonder that when we get emotionally upset the solar plexus either shuts down and we cannot digest anything or it becomes so over-stimulated that we might get stomach ulcers. All the digestive organs are conditioned by the state of the solar plexus—the stomach, liver, gall bladder, small intestine, and most of the large intestine.

Depending on our predispositions and lifestyle, disturbance of the solar plexus will manifest in different ways. Anger in one person may cause liver upsets and gallstones, and in another person may manifest as irritable bowel syndrome or ulcerative colitis.

Late-onset diabetes (usually Type II) has an inherited factor, but is becoming increasingly common, due to the level of obesity in Westerners. We can tie this problem directly back to the desire for food; this desire is a combination of energies from the sacral and solar plexus chakras.

We could say that the desire to repeat the experience of eating certain foods comes from the solar plexus and the actual sensual component of doing so from the sacral center. A lack of will from the base center can ensure that the person will go on eating and eating. Other addictions such as alcohol, and drugs like nicotine or hallucinogenic drugs, are related to the same chakra forces. The constant eating of junk food may then become the outer cause of health problems.

> *It is no wonder that when we get emotionally upset the solar plexus either shuts down and we cannot digest anything or it becomes so over-stimulated that we might get stomach ulcers. All the digestive organs are conditioned by the state of the solar plexus—the stomach, liver, gall bladder, small intestine, and most of the large intestine.*

Common health disorders relating to the solar plexus center include constipation, diarrhea, nausea, diabetes, stomach ulcers, pancreatitis, gallstones, hepatitis, irritable bowel syndrome, coeliac disease, ulcerative colitis, and Crohn's disease (inflammation of the small bowel). The outer causes of these problems may be related to poor diet and certain deficiencies, inherited predispositions, and poor lifestyle.

One of the great benefits of vitalizing and energizing the chakras above the diaphragm is for the control and right direction of the lower chakras. Note that I used the word control and not suppression. For instance, one of the main inner causes of cancer below the diaphragm is considered by some researchers to be suppression of anger. This concept is in accord with esoteric teachings that cancer may result from emotional suppression, which then causes an over-stimulation of the life principle in groups of cells, causing these cells to go out of control.

The solar plexus center is related to a number of minor centers, such as those connected with the liver, stomach, arms, legs, and the spleen. As you will see later, when discussing the healing procedures, triangles are visualized between these major and minor chakras to restore flows of energy through the digestive organs and other body parts.

The Heart Chakra: Unconditional Love

The higher counterpart or partner of the solar plexus is the heart. This chakra is found just above the diaphragm when viewed at the front of the body, and between the shoulder blades when looking at the back. Its associated tissues are the heart, arteries and veins, the breasts, and the lower lobes of the lungs. Health disorders associated with the heart chakra will be anything related to the heart and circulation, diseases of the lower lungs and of the breasts, including cancer of the lungs or breast.

The endocrine gland associated with the heart is the thymus. We know that the thymus gland produces T lymphocytes and other cells that kill foreign bodies such as bacteria, viruses, and cancer cells. This gland is therefore intimately associated with our physical immunity; in autoimmune disorders such as multiple sclerosis and lupus, I have found its energy to be disturbed.

The activation of the heart chakra provides us with psychic immunity, and this is particularly valuable in the case of healers so that they do not become subject to the transference of destructive energies from clients. When the heart becomes active, it automatically draws energy up from the solar plexus, giving control of the solar plexus chakra. This allows the person concerned to maintain stable emotions, even when all else may be in chaos.

The heart chakra, when activated, radiates unconditional and universal love. This love is distinct from the more limited and possessive type of love associated with the solar plexus that often manifests between couples, within families, and in tribal or racial groups.

Heart love is that which asks nothing for itself; true service can be seen to relate to this expression of energy. The vitalization of the centers above the diaphragm is a sign that the person is aligning with the soul, while a sense of responsibility is often coincident with this development. Such responsibility is really the ability to respond to a sensed need in our environment.

We can feel optimistic that human development is heading in the right direction if we consider the logarithmic development of altruistic groups within humanity since the second half of the twentieth century. There are now groups concerned with conserving and healing rivers, streams, oceans, and forests; groups devoted to protection of animals and children; and a general community concern with human welfare. This is an indication that the heart center within humanity as a whole is opening wide.

When considering the increase of reported autoimmune disease, we may have to pay a lot more attention to the inner causes related to the heart chakra. Have persons with these diseases suppressed their love energy in some way so that the body starts to regard its own cells and tissues as enemies? Subtle forms of healing, combined with natural remedies, have been able to reverse so-called incurable autoimmune disorders, such as multiple sclerosis and myasthenia gravis.

The minor centers associated with the heart chakra include one above the heart associated with the vagus nerve, one below the heart, and two minor centers located above the nipples. I have made an interesting observation in the iris of women who have suffered breast cancer. In the area of the iris that corresponds to the heart, I have noted a petal-shaped lesion, whereby the top layer of the iris fibers has disappeared, leaving the darker petal-shaped lesion. If one asks these women about their inner life within the last few years, there is often a deep grief involving lost love. However, this does not mean that everyone with such an iris lesion will have the other factors necessary for the manifestation of breast cancer, such as lack of antioxidants or accumulation of lymphatic toxins.

The energies that begin to flow between the solar plexus and the heart do not initially maintain an even balance. There may be joy and exuberance of the heart with, perhaps, some functional heart disorders like palpitations, contrasting at other times with imbalance in the solar plexus and resultant digestive disorders. Humanity is obviously endeavoring to come to grips and control the unruly solar plexus center. Witness the many counseling styles, psychologists and groups who are training people to own and integrate their emotions. This movement is possible because the focus is shifting from the solar plexus to the heart. We no longer need to be in danger of drowning in the sea of our emotions.

Heart Chakra Case History: Dana, 51, came to our clinic with a history of benign lung tumor. As mentioned, the disorders of the lung are associated with the heart chakra. Her current history of clinical depression was also in keeping with a heart chakra disturbance. She was on Oroxine for an underactive thyroid, a condition which also predisposes a person towards depression. She had been a poor sleeper since the death of her mother, an event that followed separation from her marriage partner.

Her diet was fairly poor and lacking in vegetables and fruit. Over some years, this would lead to an accumulation of waste in her tissues and mineral deficiencies. Indeed, her iris revealed a large accumulation of acid waste in the tissues and a congested lymphatic system. From a naturopathic viewpoint, this accumulation of waste would be the outer reason for the lung tumor, while the inner reason may well have been the grief following death and separation.

The etheric scan revealed a disturbance in the thyroid gland and an underactive heart chakra. The physical remedies I prescribed included the colloidal minerals potassium and magnesium phosphate for the depression and headaches, Vitamin E and homeopathic fucus (seaweed drops) for the thyroid, and an herbal cleansing mixture for the lymphatic congestion.

Dana and I had a discussion about her throat chakra, thyroid, and the need for creativity in her life to allow the energy to flow through the throat chakra to the thyroid. Dana was given a visualization to triangulate energies through the throat chakra and associated minor chakras at her shoulders, elbows, and hands. After two months of treatment, Dana was less depressed, had a bit more energy, and was focusing on how to bring more creativity into her life.

The final pair of chakras to consider is that of the base and the crown. They express self-will and spiritual will, respectively. Spiritual will tends to be the third and last of the three spiritual aspects we develop, so it is appropriate to consider the crown chakra last. The three pairs of chakras correlate to the three divine attributes of intelligence, love, and spiritual will and these attributes are developing gradually within humanity over thousands of years.

During the last few hundred years, this development appears to have become accelerated. Creative intelligence was the first major attribute to develop, and the Renaissance appeared to give this unfoldment a boost in many areas, including art, architecture, and in literature, through the development of the printing press. The throat chakra is associated with all creative writing, and to be able to suddenly spread the printed word to thousands of people instead of a few cultured individuals symbolizes a great expansion in the throat chakra within humanity. This movement was the external expression for the transmutation or movement of energies from sacral to throat center.

The second major attribute is love, and in the last 2000 years humanity has started to understand the meaning of love. This expression coincides with a gradual movement of energies from the solar plexus to the heart. The large changes in human consciousness after the Second World War, as mentioned in the section on the heart chakra, represented a big boost to the development of love within humanity.

The last attribute we develop is spiritual will, and its expression between individuals and nations is the will-to-good. It relates to the quality of synthesis, and this means to sense the whole. If we sense the whole we do not destroy part, whether it is a person or part of nature for, in so doing, we destroy part of ourselves. The base and crown chakras are the expression of this final transmutation from self-will (base) to spiritual will (crown), and further explanation of spiritual will is found shortly under the crown chakra.

The Base Chakra: The Will to Live

The base chakra is found below the end of the spine called the coccyx and is related to the will to be and to exist. It is sometimes called the root chakra and, as such, it relates to our family background and tree. The associated glands are the adrenals, which pour out the adrenalin when it is needed for fight, flight, or perhaps to win in a sporting situation. This chakra will be very active in the sportsman, soldier, or terrorist. It will also be very active when a person has internalized their aggression or stress; this often also manifests as high blood pressure.

Alternatively, in chronic and debilitating diseases like cancer or multiple sclerosis, the energy in the base chakra can be very low and is hardly sensed by the healer. Low blood pressure or lack of grounding involving our body energies can also manifest as a weakness in the base energy. Tissues related to this center are the spine, the adrenal glands and kidneys, ureters, and bladder, and the external genitalia. Problems and diseases of any of these tissues relate to blockages or excesses in the base chakra.

If we reflect on the function of the adrenal glands, we can see that they would have to be the endocrine glands, associated with the base center. Whether we consider the internal medulla that produces adrenaline or the cortex that produces cortisone, these substances are used for life-threatening allergies, asthma attacks, and in severe and life-threatening infections. The connection with the adrenal glands is obvious, as the main expression of the base center is the will to live and survive.

Each gland is related to the others with biochemical and hormonal processes. For instance, cortisone from the adrenal glands includes gluco-corticoids, which are related to sugar balance and, therefore, indirectly, to the pancreas. Androgens are sex hormones manufactured by the adrenals, which therefore relate to the gonads or sex organs. Hydro-corticoids from the adrenals relate to water balance, which is also governed by the antidiuretic hormone of the posterior pituitary gland. So there is a relationship in these hormonal pathways between the pancreas, adrenal glands, and the gonads.

The base chakra houses the kundalini "fire," which rises up the spine after all the chakras have become activated and vitalized. It can be raised prematurely by unwise meditation practices, such as concentrating for long periods on the lower chakras or through the use of hallucinogenic drugs; if this happens, serious health problems can result. Usually these problems manifest because the three-fold spinal channel has not been cleared of debris. This channel is composed of etheric substance and it surrounds the physical spinal cord.

In addition, there are etheric "discs" that normally separate the chakras in a protective fashion, and these must be gradually dispersed before kundalini can rise safely. If kundalini is blocked after its arousal, it can turn back and burn through the etheric web causing serious depletion of energies. The individual may be exposed to the lower levels of the astral plane before they have the ability to deal with this encounter.

Such health disturbances do not occur in individuals who lead a life balanced between study, meditation, and service. It is the slow, but sure, way, and saves time in the long run because if the chakras are forced to open before an individual is an integrated personality, the newly awakened energies can cause profound emotional disturbances that take, sometimes, lifetimes to correct.

The Crown Chakra: Spiritual Will

The higher counterpart of the base chakra is the crown, which is situated above the head and is related to spiritual will. So, in the base chakra, the will for personal survival is expressed, while the crown chakra expresses a will that is in tune with the divine will.

The crown chakra relates to the pineal gland, now known to be the leader of the endocrine "orchestra." It is a gland that governs our response to the circadian or twenty-four-hour rhythm of the body. Hormones secreted by the pineal gland include melatonin and serotonin, which are disturbed by interruptions to our circadian rhythm, such as in long plane journeys. This is why, with long and fast travel, we suffer sleep and digestive disorders and menstrual disturbances in some women.

The pineal gland is related to light changes during the 24-hour period. Melatonin production peaks between 2 A.M. and 3 A.M.—the darkest portion of the night. Some people suffer from depression in wintertime, due to light deprivation affecting the secretions from their pineal gland, and they benefit from exposure to strong full spectrum lights for a period each day. There is obviously a sensitive relationship between melatonin and serotonin production, as lack of serotonin can prevent sleep and relaxation.

In a spiritual sense, the pineal gland also responds to spiritual light, and thus meditation stimulates the pineal gland to be sensitive to light in a more subtle sense. The long-term use of melatonin may cause the side effect of suppressing the pineal's production of this hormone. A similar feedback mechanism occurs with the use of the contraceptive pill where, by giving estrogen and/or progesterone, the ovarian function of a woman is suppressed.

The crown chakra is the last to be activated, because spiritual will is a faculty not usually developed until creative intelligence and unconditional love are established. When the kundalini energy flows freely up the spinal channels, the crown chakra is fully activated and forms the light around the head depicted as the halo seen around saints and visionaries. Creative intelligence, love, and spiritual will are the three qualities that correspond to the three of the chakras above the diaphragm—the throat, heart, and crown.

The Brow Chakra: The Integrated Personality

The brow chakra, often called the "third eye," can be considered as the higher aspect of the throat center. In metaphysical teaching, we constantly find the higher mirrored in the lower—as above, so below. In several major religions, a trinity is depicted, and these aspects of deity are personified as spiritual beings that express will, love, or creative intelligence. We find this trinity reflected throughout our subtle constitution, whether we are considering the subtle bodies or the chakras.

The crown center corresponds to spiritual will, the brow center to the love-wisdom aspect, and the alta major center at the base of the skull to the intelligent creative center. These are then reflected in the three chakras above the diaphragm as head (will), heart (love), and throat (intelligence). The final reflection is below the diaphragm— solar plexus chakra (possessive love), sacral chakra (lower mind), and base chakra (selfish will). We have also discussed earlier the three attributes in connection with the three pairs of chakras.

We can work out some of the main functions of the brow center by reflecting on the functions of its related gland, the pituitary. The pituitary used to be considered the master gland of the body before the overriding aspect of the pineal was understood. Indeed, the pituitary secretes hormones that relate in a feedback mechanism with some of the five endocrine glands below the head. There is thyroid-stimulating hormone (TSH); adrenal gland-stimulating hormone (ACTH); ovarian-stimulating hormones (FSH and LH); and a growth-stimulating hormone. Hormones from the posterior part of the pituitary gland include the antidiuretic hormone, which causes reabsorption of water from the kidneys, and prolactin, which is related to milk production in nursing mothers.

In keeping with this bevy of pituitary activities, the brow center is often considered the conductor of the personality life as it gathers up and makes a synthesis of our many personality attributes. Therefore, the development of the brow chakra corresponds to personality integration, which results from gathering up the energies from the spinal chakras. Before this development, we are pulled in a number of directions by our conflicting emotions and scattered thought-life. When personality integration begins, we can start to manifest our activities with a sense of direction in whatever creative way we are moving.

For instance, an artist, instead of just painting when the mood moves her and without any particular theme in mind, might start planning an exhibition, bringing in a more disciplined work pattern, manifesting a particular theme in her work, and organizing the needed financing for the exhibition. A computer software man who is depleted by long hours and no leisure or exercise time might start working more regular hours, making time for exercise and relaxation; he may start looking for work that expresses his growing understanding of global needs in, for instance, education.

The brow chakra has the job of gathering up all our energies and focusing them in the head area to provide for a conductor effect in our life expression. This integrative effect of the brow can be selfish, so that the person concerned becomes a dynamic personality but functions as a highly ambitious person with self-centered motives. The brow chakra has a further possibility and function in its development. It can relate to the energies flowing in from the soul via the crown center; this is its more altruistic task. Thus, we could say that the brow center can look upwards or downwards—it can receive spiritual energies or respond to the heights of personality ambition.

The alignment between the pineal and pituitary gland features in the teaching of Alice Bailey[25] and Rudolf Steiner.[26] Both talk of the pituitary as representing the more earthly forces of humanity and of the pineal as relating to the activities of the soul. When the brow chakra forms an alignment correlating with the crown chakra, it becomes the distributing center for spiritual energies that can be directed wherever needed. In esoteric healing, it is the brow center that we use to send energies around the energy fields of the client. The brow center relates to the throat center in its creative aspect; to the heart center in its inclusive capacity; to the solar plexus in its imaginative aspect; and to the crown center in its capacity to help the client in relation to their soul plan.

Health problems in relation to the brow center involve the structures of the head and may include sinus congestion, headaches, eye and ear problems, nervous tension, and migraines. The associated tissues of the brow are, therefore, the eyes, ears, lower brain, sinuses, and, of course, the pituitary gland.

Health problems in relation to the brow center involve the structures of the head and may include sinus congestion, headaches, eye and ear problems, nervous tension, and migraines. The associated tissues of the brow are, therefore, the eyes, ears, lower brain, sinuses, and, of course, the pituitary gland. Therefore, other health disorders may involve parts of the body under control of the pituitary secretions. However, health disorders of the pituitary are not common.

As we start to stimulate the brow chakra in either the course of daily living or through meditation, functional problems of the eyes can develop such as astigmatism and near-sightedness. Both are caused by tensions around or within the eyeball that distort vision. Far-sightedness is caused by over-relaxation of the eye muscles and is more characteristic of older persons who find difficulty in focusing on objects or print held near to their eyes.

In terms of consciousness, we can consider the brow center as relating to the higher levels of the mind and mental level where we play with abstract and creative thought. This makes the connection with the throat chakra more obvious as the throat center is concerned with the mind, in terms of planning and scheming. The brow center receives the idea, the throat center is associated with planning, and the sacral center provides the basic energy in terms of manpower and money or supply.

We have now discussed the main seven energy centers, in terms of consciousness and their actions and connections. There are two minor centers that, although not concerned with consciousness as the major seven, are still important in terms of our health.

The Alta Major Chakra: The Nervous System

As far as I know, this center is only mentioned in the Alice Bailey teachings. The alta major is not one of the major seven but is an important minor center, as it corresponds to the throat center and therefore forms one of the major three head centers. It has an important relation to the autonomic part of the nervous system, and we use it in healing when treating the nervous system and pain. Its inflow point corresponds to the slight gap between the top of the spinal column and the skull—in other words, where the spinal cord enters the brain stem. The outflow point is on the hairline at the front. With this position on the body, it is very much concerned with balance.

The carotid "gland" is a function associated with the alta major but in terms of its position, it is an enigma. It has been suggested that this gland is connected to the fourth ventricle of the brain. Some researchers consider that the carotid gland may be associated with secreting cells in the wall of the fourth ventricle of the brain. There is no medical work as yet describing the function of the carotid gland. It may be a non-physical entity.

Health problems with the alta major are mainly related to disturbances in the autonomic nervous system and to a lack of balance between the sympathetic and parasympathetic parts of the autonomic nervous system. Such imbalance is typified in the stress suffered by individuals who are nervously affected because they push themselves too hard and who thus suppress that part of their nervous system related to relaxation, namely, the parasympathetic, including the vagus nerve. The result is that they feel very stressed because the sympathetic part of the nervous system becomes dominant and with it, hypersecretion of the adrenal glands.

Another consideration is the effect of the autonomic nervous system on digestion. If the vagus nerve or parasympathetic system is suppressed, we do not digest our food adequately, and this, in turn, leads to all sorts of digestive problems. Insomnia is another classic problem involving the alta major center. Whenever we are active, as in sport, very busy, or worrying, the alta major center diminishes in size and

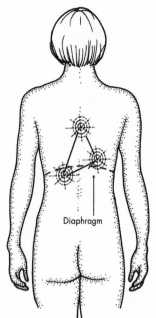

Diaphragm

FIGURE 5: THE PRANIC TRIANGLE. The pranic triangle consists of an energy center above the heart, near the diaphragm, and near the spleen.

the adrenal glands and sympathetic part of the nervous system become more active. Meditation and relaxation skills enhance the vagus nerve and the alta major then expands, stretching to its optimal size, allowing us to be more serene.

The Spleen Chakra: Reception of Prana

The spleen chakra is also not one of the major seven, but it is an extremely important center in health and healing, as it relates to our absorption of energy from the sun. I have found the spleen to be blocked in the condition known as chronic fatigue syndrome. It is situated over the spleen organ on the left-hand side, just below the diaphragm, and with two other minor centers it forms a triangle for the reception of energy called the "Pranic triangle" (see figure 5). Energy, or prana, from the Sun flows around this triangle three times almost immediately and is then distributed to all parts of the body. Even if our spleen is removed, its subtle aspect continues to function in this way through the triangle.

In our healing procedures, we visualize various triangles involving the spleen, in relation to other chakras, for the purpose of sending energy around the etheric body. (This is detailed more in the next chapter.) In Australia, medical authorities have caused the public to be paranoid about exposure to the sun. But moderate sunbathing has always been a basic part of naturopathic principles for healthy living. Even fifteen minutes of exposure of our spleen, with our back to the sun, is sufficient and can be undertaken once or twice a week, at times when the sun is not at its hottest position in the sky.

The Minor Chakras

The minor centers number over 21 (see figure 3), of which the most important are the spleen center and alta major. Some of the minor centers are associated with the digestive organs such as liver, stomach, and gall bladder. In addition, there are small centers at all the joints—even the small finger and toe joints. As you will see later when we get to the practical work in part 2, you can learn to visualize triangles between the major and minor chakras and this procedure allows energy to flow more freely through the whole body system of energies.

The minor centers are not associated with states of consciousness like the major seven centers.

Summary: The primary, secondary, and tertiary energy systems known as the chakras comprise the fundamental mechanism to be restored in esoteric healing so that energy can then flow to all the organs, tissues, blood, and cells of our body. The seven main chakras are each transmitters for a different level of consciousness; at the physical level, each is connected to an endocrine gland. They are related to each other through both hormonal and psychological pathways. As we develop psychologically and spiritually, the energies of the higher chakras gradually draw up the energies of the chakras below the diaphragm and a creative balance is established. The chakras above the diaphragm are related to development of spiritual intelligence (throat), spiritual love (heart), and spiritual will (crown).

In the next chapter, we will explore how esoteric healing techniques are used to restore energy and to balance the chakras and subtle bodies.

5 The Soul Factor in the Healing Process

By whatever name we use for it, the soul is the inner essence or center point of our being. The experience of the soul is one of peace, serenity, and understanding about ourselves in space and time. The effect of the soul on illness or disease is to bring complete ease and a sense of well-being. It is our true center of consciousness or awareness, and results from the interaction of our spirit with matter or the form through which we manifest as an individual being. The soul could be thought of as our inner essence or principle. It is indicated by the spiritual quality in our life. At the level of the soul, we are united with other souls. This is very significant for the healing process where we endeavor to act as a midwife to evoke the soul of the client.

Each of our "bodies" (physical, astral, mental) is associated with a level of consciousness. If you refer to figure 6, you will see that there are seven major planes as described by Western metaphysicians such as Blavatsky, Heindel, Steiner, and Bailey. They have described, in detail, a universe with a series of energy fields or planes whereby our consciousness gradually evolves via the lower kingdoms in nature to the human state and beyond. The soul can be understood as our center of consciousness, which develops through many lives as a human being. In a related vein, in his popular book A *Brief History of Everything*, Ken Wilbur has also developed an hierarchical view of the universe that makes useful and interesting reading.[27]

Previously, I described our physical, emotional, and mental natures as layers of the personality. We know that at times we can feel entirely separate from others at these levels of functioning,

The Seven Planes of Our Solar System
Each plane is further divided into seven subplanes in the same direction

1. Divine Plane
Deity/God/Logos/Supreme Being

- -

2. Monadic Plane
Plane of our Individualized Human Spirits

- -

3. Atmic Plane
Source of our of Spiritual Will—flows through our crown chakra

- -

4. Intuitional/Buddhic Plane
Plane of Unconditional Love—flows through our heart chakra

- -

5. Mental Plane
Plane of Thought
Higher 3 subplanes relate to abstract mind—flows via brow/ajna chakra
Our soul body resides on the third sub-plane from the top of this plane

The lower 4 subplanes express concrete or mundane thoughts
Energy from the lower mind flows through throat and sacral chakras

- -

6. Astral Plane
Plane of Desires and Feelings—flows through the solar plexus chakra

- -

7. Physical Plane
Plane of Sensation
The top four subplanes relate to our etheric body and pattern for growth
underlying our physical body—relates to the sacral chakra

The lower 3 subplanes relate to solids, liquids, and gases
These energies relate to the base chakra

FIGURE 6: THE SEVEN PLANES OF OUR SOLAR SYSTEM.

- -

despite, perhaps, making valiant efforts to communicate our feelings and thoughts. But at the level of the soul, there are no barriers at all and we have instant communication with each other. It is of interest to speculate why interpersonal boundaries disappear at the soul level.

Refer to figure 6 and note that the soul is related to the higher subplanes of the mental plane, that above it are the spiritual planes, and below it those planes relating to our personality life—lower mental, astral, and the physical plane. The lower three planes are considered to be associated with forms, and these may be physical bodies, emotions, or thoughts. Due to its position in this hierarchy, the soul can be considered as the meeting place between those levels where form, however subtle, is found and the formless planes of abstract mind, unconditional love, spiritual will, and beyond.

For our understanding of the healing process, the soul at this center point is in a unique position to transmit spiritual energies to heal the personality in any of its parts—mind, emotions, or etheric/physical body.

Reincarnation—Our Predispositions to Illness Explained

The concept that our soul gradually develops all possible human qualities through repeated lives on the lower three planes is known as reincarnation. It is a philosophy that only recently has gained wider acceptance in the West, and it is of interest that reincarnation features now in a number of recent and popular films. This is surely a sign of general public interest. According to a new study, 40% of the American population believes in reincarnation.

We cannot usually remember our past lives because we are generally so centered in our personality levels. As we gradually remove the blocks in our personality life at the emotional and mental levels, we can align with the soul more easily and memories from former lives can spontaneously manifest. Until we have soul consciousness, it is a blessing in disguise that we cannot remember some of the violent and unpleasant experiences suffered in previous lives. Having gained soul consciousness, we then have the wisdom and understanding to place any unpleasant lives in the perspective of the whole. For those who find the concept of reincarnation unbelievable,

I suggest you take a "wait and see" position, for there is no need to accept reincarnation to justify the validity of the healing techniques in this book.

Reincarnation, for me, was a logical premise to answer many of life's anomalies and inequalities that I observed. The concept resonated strongly with my intuition that we need many lives to develop all our possible talents and capacities. An increasing body of sensible and well-documented literature on personal experiences of reincarnation appears to point beyond doubt to this process as part of human development.[28] In the area of healing, reincarnation gives understanding of the differences in health and disease between one person and another. So while it is not essential for healing to accept the proposition of previous lives, it does help our acceptance of suffering, especially if disease is inherited as a predisposition.

The basic philosophy surrounding reincarnation postulates that the soul chooses parents in advance of its birth for the purpose of working out past negative situations and for developing certain skills and talents. So if, for instance, in a previous incarnation an individual abused their body through choice of a very poor diet and a lot of alcohol or drugs, perhaps their soul would attract parents who had poor health. In the present life, the person would then have the challenge to grow through having to work hard at achieving health. Or if an individual had abused their children in one life by not providing them food, they may be attracted to the challenge of being born into a family with a tubercular background, whereby they suffer from asthmatic troubles and have trouble assimilating minerals such as calcium.

The Chain of Healing

For our healing purposes, we should review again the basic equation of how spirit and matter produce consciousness and observe that it manifests as three attributes: spirit, soul, and body. Thus, soul is the middle or consciousness aspect, while body is understood to include the subtle bodies of mind, emotions and the physical body. As stated earlier, in the subtle healing process we endeavor to invoke the soul to flow through the mechanism of mind, emotions, and physical body via the chakra system. We also need to consider again the flow of energy from the soul as a chain that goes as follows:

Soul → mental body → feeling body
(astral)→ energy body (etheric) → physical body.

I mentioned earlier that there are chakras at the mental, astral, and etheric levels and that these three layers of chakras can best be thought of as interpenetrating one another, rather than as being on "top" of each other. One of the most interesting findings in my healing practice has been that quite often the physical problem of a client may be removed, but the energy pattern continues as a chaotic and circulating disturbance. In other words, the energy of a particular organ has ceased to flow harmoniously to other organs and tissues and has formed a "short circuit" in the body. When we align with the soul, balance the chakras, and triangulate energies between chakras and organs, harmony is restored. So what does triangulating the energies mean?

> A *unique technique of esoteric healing is the triangulation of energies, as presented by Alice Bailey. When we visualize a triangle as three points involving any of the chakras and organs, energy flows more freely and blockages or energy disturbances can be removed.*

The Triangulation of Energies

A unique technique of esoteric healing is the triangulation of energies, as presented by Alice Bailey. A triangle involves two points plus a third mediating point. When we visualize a triangle as three points involving any of the chakras and organs, energy flows more freely and blockages or energy disturbances can be removed. Most disease and illness involve a stasis or blockage of energy in one or more parts of the human system at physical, emotional, and mental levels. Stasis at the mental level will eventually filter down to the emotional and physical bodies. Conversely, a blockage from inflammation, drugs, viruses, or other causes in the physical body will work back up into the energy body where it stays, even when the physical factors are removed.

You may wonder how visualizing a triangle between the chakras of a person can have a healing effect. The process of esoteric healing is based on our alignment with the soul plus the flow of energy following thought. The concept of *energy follows thought* is used in many self-help programs where participants are taught to visualize what they wish to achieve or receive in life. Creative visualization is taught by many meditation teachers and is the subject of many books. In relation to the healing process of ourselves or another person, it has been found that the connection of three points by imagining light between those points—creative visualization—causes a flow of healing energy. This is augmented by means of the preparatory alignment with the soul (see below).

It is of interest that many clients *feel* the energy moving in the areas of their body where the healer's attention is focused. In the practice of esoteric healing, we allow energy in the client to normalize through soul alignment, rather than to imagine pushing energy around the client. The first law of healing in the Bailey treatise on the subject is that the "art of the healer resides in releasing the soul," so the initial alignment process is all-important.

Note that when I describe the healing process in terms of chakra balancing and visualization of triangles, it is always preceded by alignment with the soul despite the fact I may not always mention this process each time. The connection of the healer with her soul and with that of the client allows the experience of peace and serenity for the client during the healing process.

I am frequently faced with a client who has taken hormones such as estrogen or cortisone, or perhaps antibiotics, over a long period. Despite visiting me some time after cessation of taking drugs, the client's etheric body is still congested in certain parts. This is because our subtle mechanisms become changed under the influence of the virus or drug and are not automatically restored to their normal pulsation of energies. Introducing healthy energy by a triangulation of energies appears to restore this energy flow in the part concerned. I find the physical natural therapies work faster and more effectively when the etheric body is pulsating normally.

Making the Soul Alignment

Before we get to the details of how to triangulate energies with chakras and organs, I need to explain how the healer makes a basic

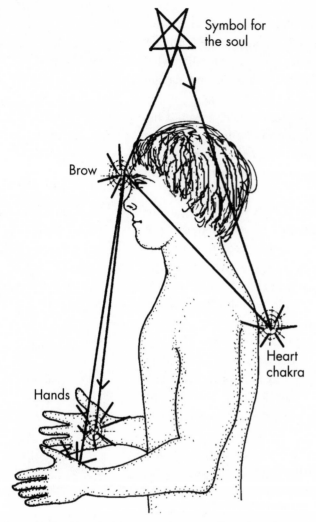

Symbol for the soul

Brow

Heart chakra

Hands

FIGURE 7: THE HEALER'S ALIGNMENT. The energy flows from the soul to the heart chakra and then to the brow chakra, then from the brow to the client via the hands. This soul, heart, head, and hands alignment protects the healer, because the energy flows through the heart before going to the head. Note that even though the symbol for the soul is placed above the head, the soul potentially pervades the energy field.

alignment between her soul and the client. This approach to healing presupposes that the healer is doing regular meditation with the aim of aligning with his soul. (For an example of a suitable meditation for soul alignment, see appendix 1.) Usually we have the client sitting in a comfortable position in the chair or, if indisposed, they can lie down.

1. Gently place your hands on the client's shoulders.

2. Imagine linking to your own soul, the client's soul, and with the source of all healing.

3. Ask that healing take place according to the plan of the soul for that person.

4. Link your soul, heart center, and brow center and visualize your hands as an extension of this triangle. Wait for a sense of the energy flowing along this pathway of soul, heart, brow, and hands, and then remove your hands and begin to balance the client's chakras (see figure 7).

In this procedure, two triangles have been made, which involve the preparation of the healer as she approaches the healing procedure. The first triangle is the healer's soul, client's soul, and source of all healing; the second triangle is the healer's soul, heart, and brow center. The client takes a passive role during the procedure. Clients can help to restore their own etheric energies with meditation and visualization.

Visualization—Seeing in a New Way

Visualization is related to our imagination, but the capacity to visualize does not mean that we have to see something in front of our eyes as if we are looking at a picture. A few clairvoyant people can do this but, in healing, we mainly work with the sense of touch. To visualize successfully, we only need to have a clear idea and feeling about something. In other words, we see something in our mind's eye. Stop reading now and remember an enjoyable event during the last month. It may involve seeing, touching, hearing, smelling, tasting, or all five faculties, but it's an *inner* seeing. This is the type of visualizing most commonly used.

In the healing process, we visualize triangles this way: imagine lines of light connecting chakras and organs, then fill this triangle with light. You do not have to see the chakras or triangles; just postulate they are there. Because the sense of touch is that most closely involved with healing, I will now discuss this sense in relation to diagnosing and scanning the chakras.

Scanning and Sensing the Chakras

Most people develop a sense of etheric touch very easily when learning to heal. This skill could be called clairsentience or clear feeling (clairvoyance means clear seeing and clairaudience means clear hearing). We have a number of minor chakras on the hands, including in the palm, and this is the main one used for diagnosing and healing. But we also have minor chakras on the fingertips and at the joints of each finger and thumb. We need to activate our hand chakras when starting to study esoteric healing methods.

Excellent exercises for activating the palms and the secondary chakra system are outlined in *Astral Dynamics* by Robert Bruce.[29] In fact, Bruce makes the point that for spiritual development it is good to activate the secondary system before working with the main chakras. It is a point worth considering, because many healers are not too healthy themselves. It seems logical that for health we need energy to flow between all the chakras, and it may be that concentrating on only the major chakras draws too much energy away from other body systems, especially if there are blockages among the minor ones.

Bruce describes exercises in which we use an imaginary pair of arms to energize, brush, and circulate energy through all the minor chakras of our hands, toes, and limbs. In my seminars, I ask people to first sense the energy between their palms while gently moving the hands in and out from each other with palms facing each other. Most people after a few moments feel a sense of elasticity between the hands or tingling, heat, or cold. Students then pair off and I ask one person to draw a pattern with a fingertip on the palm of the other person while holding their finger at least twelve inches away. The recipient holds both palms upwards with eyes shut and has to guess which palm is being activated and, if possible, describe the pattern. It is surprising the high percentage of persons who get this correct.

Exercise for Sensing the Chakras: This sensing exercise is to see if you can sense your own chakras with your hand held some inches away from the body. Start by holding your hand in the area of the solar plexus. Gently move the hand towards and away from your body until you sense the same elastic sensation as between the hands earlier. Depending on how energized you feel on a particular day, the strength of the energy will vary. Try another chakra, such as the sacral center (just above the pubic bone) or the heart center, and note the sensations.

Exercise to Sense Your Partner's Chakra: Now you are ready to sense the chakra on a partner. Start by doing the soul alignment described on page 72. Then move to the left-hand side of your partner and take up a comfortable position by kneeling on a cushion. Place your right hand about twelve inches behind their spine just above their waistline and place your left hand twelve or eighteen inches in front. Gently move the hands in and out but do not go too close to the body. After a while, you will note the energy flow of their solar plexus. Is the energy flow the same on both sides of the body? During this, realign several times with your own energy flow of soul, head, heart, and hands (see figure 7).

It is useful to also check the size of the chakras from side to side before and after the healing. To do this, stand in front of the person and gently move your hands in an accordion fashion while thinking of the chakra. This is a different measurement than when you balance the chakras as, in that case, you are sensing the energy flowing through the chakra from front to back in terms of its spin. Now you are sensing size.

As an individual develops their personality and starts to bring in soul energies, the chakras will expand considerably. Yet they also shrink with exhaustion and, as mentioned very often before the healing, one or more chakras will be found to be smaller than others on the same person. Overall, I have found the size of the chakras, when measured from side to side, varies from five to fifteen inches.

You can also note a further triangle in this practice session between your brow chakra and your two hands. Imagine energy gently flowing between these three points as it passes through the solar plexus of the client. When you experience a balance between both your hands, move to the sacral chakra, situated in a line just above the pubic bone, and repeat the process.

After balancing the sacral center, this may be a good time to start practicing a simple series of triangles related to the sacral center. I call them the grounding triangles. It is especially useful to visualize these triangles on individuals who have problems grounding their energies. Such people cannot, metaphorically, keep their feet on the ground. They may be unable to materialize ideas or perhaps unable to use money wisely; remember that the handling of money relates to the sacral chakra.

As mentioned, when we triangulate energies in the healing process, we are connecting three points—two opposing points and a mediating point—and this triangulation of energy allows the energy to flow harmoniously. To carry out this process, we align our brow center with one point—perhaps the sacral center of the client—and then use the hands to align with their other two points. We then visualize lines of light connecting the three points and we imagine filling the triangle with light. In other words, we are using three chakras in our own body, the brow and two hand chakras, to align with three points on the client. It does not matter which points on ourselves align with those of the client, but we usually align our brow center to the main chakra under consideration on the client, in this case, the sacral center.

We now visualize three sets of triangles, one after the other, on

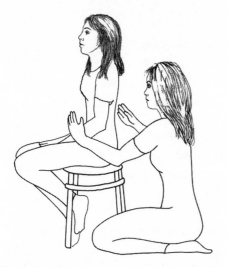

FIGURE 8A: BALANCING THE SACRAL CHAKRA. After the initial alignment, a triangle is formed between the brow center and the hands of the healer, and the energy is then balanced between the back and front of the sacral center. A similar procedure is enacted for the other chakras up the spine.

the client. These triangles are sacral and two minor hip chakras; sacral and two minor knee ones; and sacral and two minor ones on the feet (see figure 8c). Remember—you do not actually have to see the triangles in front of you to succeed in this healing work. Just imagine the triangles in your mind's eye and your energy will follow your thought. After a while, you will have a sense of when the triangle is working and you can move on to the next one. Spending a minute on each triangle is usually ample time. Just as you can measure the flow of energies of the major triangles, you can assess the flow of energy in the minor chakras. There should be a normal pulsation and movement of energies in all major and minor chakras, and also in all body organs and tissues.

When thinking about these chakras on the hips and legs, I often find in cases of arthritis that

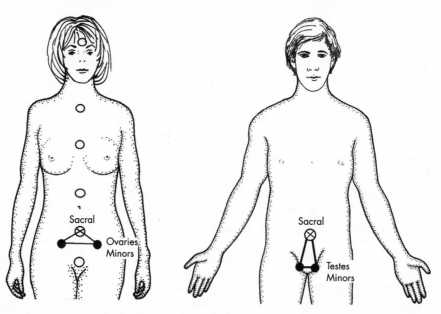

FIGURE 8B: THE SACRAL AND GROUNDING CHAKRAS. The sacral triangles are used for problems with the reproductive organs and especially for ovarian and uterine disorders in the female. These triangles are also used for infertility and sexual problems.

the energies are blocked in some of the joints related to these minor chakras. After the healing process, the energies begin to flow again normally. We often find blockages in the other minor chakras associated with the sacral center, such as those associated with the ovaries and testes. In a woman with infertility, the ovarian minor chakras are often shut down, so it is very useful to make a triangle between the sacral center and the ovaries. These are all simple triangles that you can practice on yourself and others (see figure 8b).

To practice healing yourself, imagine that you are looking at yourself in a mirror or alternatively, that you are sitting sideways on your lap. Balance each chakra as if you had another person sitting on your lap. The various triangles can then be added. Later, I will describe the balancing of the remaining spinal chakras and the use of further triangles.

To summarize the process, the overriding factor here is alignment with our inner essence or soul. Throughout the healing process, we try to maintain this alignment of soul, heart, head, and hands. If our mind wanders, we re-make the alignment from time to time of soul, heart, head, and hands, and then go back to the chakra or triangle in question. It is often helpful to have gentle music in the background as an additional focus, as this tends to counteract the effect of human voices, barking dogs, and other sounds in the environment. It also is relaxing for the client.

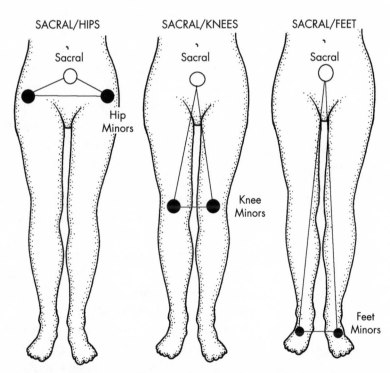

FIGURE 8C: THE GROUNDING TRIANGLES. The grounding triangles bring the energies down through the legs and feet so that excess energy is removed and the individual is literally more grounded in all their activities. It also removes congestion in the pelvis and energy blocks in the hips and legs.

The second main factor is that we visualize linking up with the soul of the client so that the healing will proceed according to the plan for their soul. If there is some strong karmic reason why they cannot be healed totally in a physical sense, they can still experience the peace and serenity that comes from soul alignment. I remember one elderly man whose daughter brought him from forty miles away. He was so weak with terminal bone cancer that he had to lie down in the back of the car throughout the journey. The interesting fact about this man was that he classed himself as an atheist, but he liked to have the healing, because he experienced great peace from it. During the healing his daughter remained in the room and she felt helped with respect to his imminent passing.

Healing and Death

These thoughts bring to mind an important reason for contacting the soul in the healing process. There is a large role for healers in preparing people for dying, so that death can be accompanied by joy in the preparation for the next phase of the soul's journey. The enormous increase of literature dealing with near-death experiences and what lies beyond has served to educate humanity to the fact that death should not be feared. But for many people it is still a terrible fear. By bringing the soul into the healing process, we can give a person the sense of peace and joy that comes from soul contact.

It is the soul that decides when our personality has run its life course. However, modern medicine often prolongs the physical body beyond its own capacity for reasonable function and can thus thwart the soul impulse. On the other hand, perhaps this is an argument against euthanasia. I am inclined to think that when a certain percentage of humanity recognizes and works with their soul purpose, the question of euthanasia will be resolved, as will the question of prolongation of life beyond healthy function.

When the majority of the population understands and/or experiences that death is not the end to our journey, then our attitude to health and disease will change. In fact, we must begin to understand that healing the physical body is not always the reason for undertaking the healing process. More important is the healing of the psyche by means of calling in the soul. Very often, the healing ultimately takes place by means of a peaceful death.

The Soul and the Meaning of Life

One of the drawbacks of New Age literature has been the excesses of guru-centered writings and workshops, charging large sums of money for meditation and healing techniques to transport one into bliss and the "higher" realms. This has inhibited the study of more serious and sensible literature by more conservative persons. However, by whatever name the soul or higher self is known, the abundance of personal experience by intelligent and well-educated persons now gives great hope that there are higher forces guiding our destiny.

The soul is measured by the quality of our life. In many cases, disease can be seen as an opportunity for the individual to gain more understanding about the meaning of life. As soon as they start to ask "why me?" there is the opportunity and potential for growth. Thus, we often hear of cancer sufferers who have accepted their disease as a challenge say that they would not have missed this opportunity to bring more quality into their life through greater understanding. It seems to be a fact of life on our planet that we learn by suffering. Why should this be so? Why does it take a major life crisis to make us appreciate life? Why, given the beauty and biological diversity of our planet, are most people still mainly concerned with material values?

Mention of the soul cycling around the lower three planes from life to life has been postulated as a way to account for how we acquire attributes and qualities for the soul. But life on other planets may not necessarily include a physical level for this evolution. It is possible that on many planets human life only descends to the etheric level, and the souls evolving there may never have or need a physical body, except if they wish to materialize for the purpose of contacting individuals on our planet. There is no reason why consciousness cannot evolve through the various levels without having a biological and physical form for its basis.

However, because our planet has developed physical forms as expressed in the various kingdoms in nature, we have a greater challenge than if, for instance, our consciousness was centered on a planet where the lowest level of expression was etheric. In that case, we would have an energy body but no physical body. Perhaps our planet is a unique experiment of a creator to see how humanity can cope with physical forms.

The point I am coming to here is that, in terms of health and disease as experienced in the twenty-first century, large sections of humanity have become identified with physical and material values. The underlying soul energies thus have no opportunity to keep a healthy etheric pattern to form the mold for physical growth.

The point I am coming to here is that, in terms of health and disease as experienced in the twenty-first century, large sections of humanity have become identified with physical and material values. The underlying soul energies thus have no opportunity to keep a healthy etheric pattern to form the mold for physical growth. So we have become so identified with our physical body and possessions that we have forgotten our higher self and source. It is only when our physical form or body is threatened with destruction (often through poor lifestyle) that we start to question the meaning of life. Sometimes, this search follows total loss of physical support in the form of home, money, possessions, or a precious relationship.

But the positive side of the coin is that our planet has a greater inherent beauty in its diversity of biology than has yet been observed on any other planet. So, once we have learned to align with the soul, we can bring spirit into matter, and when a certain proportion of humanity functions this way, perhaps our planet can be healed in many ways. I am suggesting here that individual healing is part of a much wider healing process that is starting to take place on our planet as increasing numbers of people nurture and heal vegetable, animal, and human forms.

The invocation of the soul in the healing process as described here can be seen as a fundamental need, not just for the individual, but also for the planet. Healing needs to be both inner and outer. For this reason, the basic natural therapies of vitamins, minerals, and herbs are just as important as calling in the soul. Many esoteric therapies ignore the physical needs of the body and address only half of the equation. I find in practice that the two sides of the coin, inner and outer healing, are essential in most cases.

Summary: The essence of the healing process is to contact the soul and to be able to invoke this central factor from within the client to flow through the chain of mind, feelings, energy body, and physical body. There is a sensing process in which the therapist will know where the disturbances are in the client. Then there is an alignment process, followed by visualization involving the triangulation of energies between the chakra, minor chakras, and physical organs. Through an ability to contact our healing essence of soul, we can prepare ourselves and others for a peaceful death and gain meaning, meanwhile, about our place in life.

In the next chapter, we explore the various categories of disease by looking in detail at two cornerstones of natural therapy and healing: vitality and toxic waste. Toxic waste can accumulate in the body from both inner and outer factors—in other words, from our inner and outer diet. Similarly, our vitality or energy is conditioned by many factors. So we will be looking at immunity both from an inner and outer perspective, and we will explore the three stages of disease: the acute, sub-acute, and chronic.

We need to keep in mind the soul connection when even considering the three stages of disease. The further away we move from our inner alignment, the more likely it is that a disease process can move in the direction of chronic ill health. Recognizing the healing energies underlying our physical form also has wider implications for the healing of the planet in many respects. We are challenged to consider why we have tended to forget our spiritual source and to keep visualizing the wide effects for healing when the majority of human beings align with their soul energies.

6 Stages of Disease As Related to Toxins and Vitality

The two pillars of naturopathic treatment for 150 years have been the improving of vitality and the eliminating of waste from the body. Toxins come from external and internal causes (see figure 1 in chapter 1), and the nerve toxins caused by negative emotions can rival anything toxic we take in from the environment in air, water, food, or chemicals.

However, our level of vitality is perhaps a more significant factor than the level of toxins. Vitality comes from, among other things, positive emotions, sunlight, whole foods, and pure water. Regular meditation can greatly enhance our vitality through bringing in soul energies. All the aforementioned factors condition our etheric or energy body, that part of our constitution underlying all the physical organs and tissues (see chapter 3).

The etheric body conditions the electromagnetic field that interfaces between our etheric and physical bodies. This field carries information for growth and repair. If our vitality or basic energy is high, then the body tends to throw off toxins. As vitality lessens due to poor diet, lack of sunlight, chemical overload, electromagnetic stress, or advancing age, toxins accumulate and eventually interfere with the functioning of body processes through the development of chronic disease. We will shortly follow this process through the three stages of disease—acute, sub-acute, and chronic.

Both the level of vitality and degree of toxic overload in the body can be very quickly estimated through a study of the iris. This form of diagnosis is commonly used by natural therapists. Acupuncturists usually assess vitality and organ function through the pulse diagnosis and both acupuncturists and naturopaths examine the tongue for a quick indication of toxic levels, but the iris is more indicative of conditions that have been present for many years. Iris diagnosis was pioneered by Dr. Ignatz Von Peckzely during the years between 1840 and 1850 in Budapest, Hungary.

Iris Diagnosis and Vitality

Dr. Von Peckzely researched iris markings after noticing a black spot appeared in the eye of an owl after it broke a leg. He systematically correlated organ disease with sections of the iris and linked general discolorations of the iris color with particular toxins and drugs. The twentieth-century American naturopath Bernard Jensen, N.D., became the most famous pioneer in iridology, and during his long career he popularized the method of diagnosis and taught thousands of therapists via his publications and specialized equipment.[30]

Over the years, I have found iris diagnosis to be a very good general guide to the inherited vitality of a person and to the accumulation of toxins in their system. The tongue, ear, and hand can also be used for diagnosis, but the iris is superb because it has a rich blood and nerve supply, and its radial fibers lend themselves to an evaluation with mathematical precision. Precision is important when looking at the position for organs and tissues in the body (see iris chart, figure 9). When you look at the iris of a baby, it is usually shiny and clear, with all the fibers close together and no toxic markings. This iris picture indicates excellent vitality. It is disappointing to see the changes that occur in the iris over the years with poor diet, pollution, immunizations, and stress.

The iris can reveal the presence of toxicity that has both outer and inner causes. So occasionally, we encounter a person with a very good diet but with so much anger, grief, or depression that the iris reveals they have a very acid constitution. Inherited and metabolic factors also play a part. Sometimes, I see a mother and daughter with very similar discolorations in their iris indicating that they have accumulated much uric and lactic acid in their tissues due to inherited

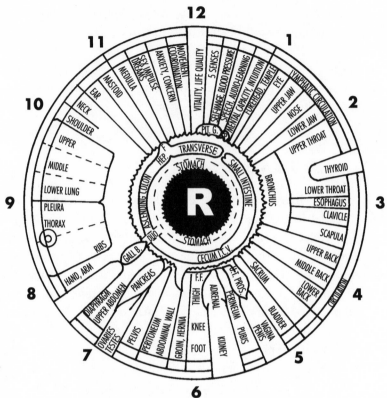

FIGURE 9: THE IRIS MAP. This map shows the segments of the iris that correspond to the different organs in the body. Note that these are the positions when facing the other person.

Adapted from iris chart in *Iridology* by Dorothy Hall (Australia: Viking, Penguin, 1989).

metabolic errors, despite a reasonably good diet. Such clients often manifest rheumatism or arthritic tendencies as they age.

The Three Stages of Disease

Naturopaths understand disease to progress in roughly three stages, namely, acute, sub-acute, and chronic, and that these stages correlate to the state of one's vitality and toxicity. We have all observed the fantastic vitality that a young, healthy baby demonstrates—the bright and darting eyes, the quick movements, the alertness. It is depressing to see the same child seven years later with nervous irritability, eczema or asthma, and mucus running continuously from its nose. The mother may have brought the child to our clinic because of severe ear infections that arise every time a cold develops.

On questioning, we may find that the child is very picky with its food and refuses vegetables and most other foods. So Mum tries to

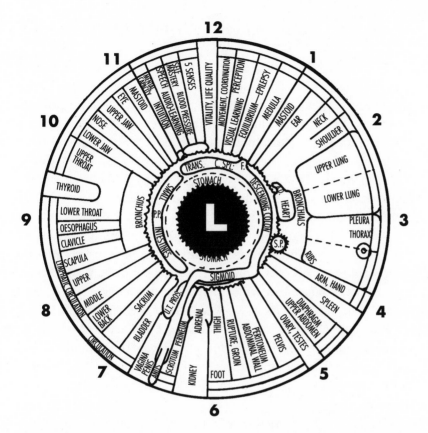

make up this loss with lots of milk and gives in to the child's demands for biscuits and sweets to "keep his energy up." We then have a vicious circle of poor diet causing lack of appetite and further accumulation of waste that the young body tries to eliminate through mucus. Each time a virus is encountered, there will be severe secondary infections because of the accumulated waste, in the same way that flies are attracted to a rubbish tin.

Acute Disease

So what has happened to the healthy baby? When our vitality is high and toxicity levels are low, we have good health, and if an infection is encountered, it usually runs a short course with no long-term side effects. When body energies are good, our inherent vitality tends to bring waste to the surface, and the body responds to a passing virus by creating fever that burns up the toxins. They are then transformed into substances that are excreted by the bowels, skin, lungs, or kidneys.

This concept has been proved to me over many years of observing how clients who previously suffered severe infections from upper respiratory viruses have reduced the number and severity of their infections after naturopathic treatment. Other examples are persons with a tendency to gastrointestinal infections or cystitis who have experienced increased resistance to their infections following naturopathic treatment. Studies using vitamin C indicate that the number and severity of colds per year are reduced by taking doses of at least 1 gram of vitamin C daily.

We could say again that the severity of the infection is related to the level of toxins and degree of vitality in the person. This appears to be why some people in an epidemic escape infection, even when close to those infected, or why others suffer it severely.

Also contrast the practices of mainstream medicine with the use of natural supplements such as vitamin C[31] and selected herbs[32] to promote immunity, resolve infection, and to keep the immune system in balance. The use of esoteric healing has a role in resolving energy blocks that relate to poor organ function and, indirectly, to poor immunity.

The acute stage of disease may include all or some of the following factors: redness, heat, fever, and/or swelling. Eczema, boils, and abscesses are typical here; sore throats, reaction to insect stings, and the initial inflammation associated with colds and flu before manifestation of mucus are further examples. Common childhood infections such as chicken pox, rubella, measles, and mumps also fall into this category, provided that there are no further complications. If there are complications after having a virus like measles, such as ear infections or, at worst, encephalitis (inflammation of the brain), then, from a naturopathic viewpoint, this disease process indicates that the child had a toxic body *before* the infection.

Acute Disease Case History: Ann was a 39-year-old nurse administrator involved with accreditation of nursing homes. She also had training in the area of herbal medicine, but occasionally visited me for health crises. Her iris revealed that her body had accumulated a lot of waste, chiefly in the lymphatic system. She had visited me earlier for eczema on the feet. This problem cleared up in two months with a herbal mixture containing equal parts of red clover, catmint, cat's claw, burdock, and poke root; homeopathic toning drops for the liver and lymphatic system; the tissue salts iron phosphate and potassium chloride for the stages of inflammation of the eczema; and potassium and magnesium phosphate for the "nerve rings" in her iris.

Eighteen months later, Ann was subject to a lot of stress at work and allowed her healthy diet to degenerate so that she was indulging in more junk food than normal. She made an appointment to seek relief from what she described to me as a boil. I asked to inspect the boil and was concerned to see an area of hard inflammation of at least two square inches that I would have described as an abscess rather than a boil. It was situated under the right costal region (below the ribs).

She was already on an herbal mixture, but it was not a suitable prescription for this type of problem. I added two herbs to stimulate the immune system, cat's claw and burdock, plus the liver and lymphatic homeopathic drops to which had been added a homeopathic antidote to staphylococcal infection. In addition, I gave Ann a tablet containing high amounts of vitamin B complex plus multiminerals. I included the tissue salt calcium sulfate. The effect of these remedies is to resolve the infection via the lymphatic system rather than by "ripening" the abscess. This latter process encourages the infection to come to the surface, where it can be lanced to expel the pus. I chose not to pursue this course with Ann, preferring to resolve the situation by cleansing the whole lymphatic system and encouraging her lymph glands to drain out the toxicity.

Ann was very sensitive to subtle energies, and during the esoteric healing she experienced her spiritual guides assisting with the healing. During this healing, I focused on helping to move out the toxins that had caused the abscess by doing the lymphatic drainage process. This is a technique whereby, after balancing the chakras, we use a gentle wafting movement of the hands to move the toxins from the affected area to the minor chakras near the clavicle bones (collarbone). This is a technique that needs to be learned in a professional workshop situation. All these movements are done from a distance of a few feet, and it never ceases to amaze me how powerful these subtle techniques can be.

The abscess cleared up in a few days and Ann did not need to return. It is always difficult for me to say what helps the most, the natural medicines or the subtle healing. I prefer to think of them as complementary. As for the cause, in this case, Ann provided the outer cause by her poor diet for a body already suffering an accumulation of toxic waste. The inner factor was the stress with her work, and as the abscess appeared very close to the gallbladder, perhaps it was the emotion of irritability and frustration with people involved with the accreditation process of nursing homes that governed the *site* of the abscess. For example, anger and irritation are traditionally associated with the hepatic system (liver and gallbladder) in Chinese medicine.

> *The result of suppressing acute disease is that the vitality of the body is somewhat diminished and toxins sink deeper into the tissues. One no longer has the energy to manifest a fever, but the body tries to eliminate toxic waste by means of a continual mucus discharge from the nose, throat, chest, or vagina.*

Sub-Acute Disease

The medical model since the 1950s has encouraged people to suppress fevers with salicylates (aspirins) and to treat infections with antibiotics. Despite the fact that most colds and flu infections are self-limiting processes and cannot be cured with antibiotics, it was still standard procedure until recently to give antibiotics to everyone consulting a medical clinic for these infections. We now know how resistant bacteria have become to antibiotics, and now some doctors are reluctant to use these drugs so freely. However, a sociological factor has entered into the picture, because patients often expect to receive a prescription for drugs when they see a doctor, and on occasion, they almost demand it.

The result of suppressing acute disease is that the vitality of the body is somewhat diminished and toxins sink deeper into the tissues. One no longer has the energy to manifest a fever, but the body tries to eliminate toxic waste by means of a continual mucus discharge from the nose, throat, chest, or vagina. Occasionally, mucus is discharged continually with the bowel actions. Unfortunately, again the medical treatment is usually to give antibiotics, despite the fact that, in many cases, the mucus is not sent to a laboratory to see if there are infective organisms present. Antibiotics further suppress the energy and immunity of the body, so toxins sink deeper into the body.

Chronic Disease

In this stage, there is both lack of vitality and the accumulation of toxins. From a naturopathic perspective, all chronic disease falls into this category. Examples are severe arthritis, chronic asthma, all kinds of severe gastrointestinal disturbances, like diverticulitis (inflammation of bowel pockets), stomach ulcers, and all the autoimmune disorders (described in the next chapter), including ulcerative colitis, multiple sclerosis, and rheumatoid arthritis.

The final stage may well be something as severe as cancer, but I find that with most chronic diseases there are deep-seated psychic disturbances that have been present for years such as suppressed anger, grief, and depression. These emotions affect the subtle constitution and immunity, and tend to allow inherited predispositions to manifest.

The interesting factor here is that inherited predispositions often indicate that the individual has started life with a body already in the sub-acute stage, due to a chronic problem manifesting earlier in the family tree. So although, from the perspective of the parent, their child was healthy for the first twenty-five years of life, a chronic disease process is often smoldering beneath the surface, waiting to be triggered by poor nutrition, psychological stress, or environmental pollution.

The Retracing Phenomenon

Over the years, I have observed that, with the correct treatment, chronic and sub-acute diseases can be retraced backwards through earlier disorders experienced by the client. A common example is the alternation in clients between asthma and eczema.

Asthma, in its moderate form as suffered by many children, often follows an earlier history of eczema, which is an example of an acute disease. It has been my experience that when eczema is suppressed, either by diminished vitality in the child or through the use of cortisone, asthma commonly develops. During the course of naturopathic treatment, the situation often reverses and the eczema returns, and if the skin condition is correctly treated, the asthma does not return. Although the medical profession would interpret both eczema and asthma as Type 1 sensitivities of the immune system, eczema is obviously less life-threatening than asthma. Another example, though less common, is a severely arthritic patient who will go back to experiencing a chronic mucus discharge and then, finally, when that is resolved, a skin eruption will appear so that all three stages of disease are experienced.

Sometimes the retracing will take a different form and go from the more important organ systems to those not quite so important for everyday survival. For instance, the immune system, lymphatic system, or digestive system could be considered more immediately important than the reproductive system. Hence, in a client with problems in these areas, the reproductive area may be the last to move back to health. Conversely, as mentioned earlier, I have noted that for many women, as soon as they get stressed and below par with their general health, libido is the first thing to disappear.

Case Study that Shows Retracing: Fay's case was a good example of how the body sometimes retraces to health through different organ systems. In this case, her digestive system was corrected first and then the reproductive system, as this latter system is less important for the overall health. This is an interesting case because so many organ systems were involved, and both naturopathic and esoteric treatment were continued for many months.

Fay, 33, had a high-pressure job that included traveling throughout Southeast Asia to conduct training sessions for employees of a large oil company. She first came to my clinic with a history of repeated viruses occurring over many months, as well as exhaustion and headaches, a tendency to constipation, and endometriosis. Antibiotics had not helped her infections, and specialized gynecological treatment had not helped her reproductive system. My energy scanning indicated disturbances of her liver, small intestine, large bowel, ovaries, uterus, and right bronchus.

I started treatment to improve her digestion and energy. I gave her an herbal mixture for her digestion, containing meadowsweet, angelica, St. Mary's thistle, and marshmallow root; colloidal potassium and magnesium phosphate for her nerves; and potassium sulfate for her infected mucus. Her digestion rapidly improved, and then we worked more on her reproductive system. I gave her colloidal calcium phosphate to help her painful periods and a different mixture for her reproductive organs. This mixture included viburnum, lady's mantle, shepherd's purse, and meadowsweet. Fay stayed on this mixture for several years, and it helped resolve her endometriosis and painful, heavy periods.

Fay received esoteric healing each month, and after the chakra balancing and vitality triangles, she had other triangles for digestion, sacral balance and grounding, and for her endocrine system and for lymphatic drainage. On her second visit, energy scanning indicated that the bronchials had cleared, but the small and large intestines, ovaries, and uterus were still disturbed. In other words, Fay's body was attending to the immune system first, rather than the ovaries and uterus.

On Fay's third visit, the energy disturbances of the ovaries appeared to have disappeared, according to my energy scan, but she continued to have intermittent digestive and reproductive disturbances for some months. Both naturopathic and esoteric procedures were continued. After a period of about a year, Fay remained well, and she subsequently visited only every couple of months.

Fay talked about starting a family, and I concentrated on her reproductive system, as her ovaries had become disturbed again, giving rise to "spotting" before periods. I gave her an extract of wild yam, as a skin cream, to balance her hormones. (In the later chapter on hormones, fertility and hormonal balance are explored more fully. In this case study, I am mainly concerned to indicate the natural wisdom of the body as it repairs itself in the most important areas *first* in its journey back to health.)

In summary, the most interesting outcome for Fay was that her immune system remained healthy for years, and she only suffered the occasional mild respiratory infection. Her period pains have also been absent for more than two years. She has chosen to remain on a maintenance dose of supplements, and has learned to boost these with extra vitamin C, echinacea, and mineral tissue salts when suffering a virus. This can prevent secondary infections following a viral attack from developing.

Still, there are times when a client presents with such an overwhelming dose of toxins that one wonders whether retracing back to health can ever take place. David was such a case (see below). These individuals have usually been exposed to internal and external chemicals for many years, and this may be compounded by constitutional factors. However, it is surprising what can be achieved if the client perseveres for a few years and is prepared to put aside the requisite funds for such treatment. During this time, they are educated to change their lifestyle to include an emphasis on whole foods in the diet.

Case Study on Elimination of Toxins: David had suffered one of the worst accumulations of toxins I had ever witnessed. At age 24, he visited me after a car crash, in which he suffered a smashed ankle. He had a history of allergies spanning ten years and had spent thousands of dollars with the leading allergy specialist in Melbourne (Australia) without any improvement in his condition. His symptoms included fatigue, severe headaches, poor memory and concentration, panic attacks, abdominal pains, hives, recurrent boils on all areas of his body, and allergies from perfumes, solvents, disinfectants, and hydrocarbons. He had to use a face mask to filter his air intake whenever traveling outside his home, even in places like libraries.

His toxic overload began *in utero*, as his mother had lupus and was apparently heavily medicated during her pregnancy with David. She later died, when comparatively young, from this condition. David did not speak until he was four years old. He now has a good outlook on life and is concerned with conservation and ecological issues. He organizes the movement in Melbourne each year to protect and rescue injured ducks during the annual duck-shoot in the State of Victoria. Some of his toxins originated from work he used to do with gem-crafting, in which a very toxic oil product is used in the cutting of gems.

David's iris revealed the extent of his toxicity. There was an overlay of brown on his normal color of green; also visible were heavy lymphatic markings and signs that his nervous system had been stretched to the limit. The energy scan revealed disturbances in his lymphatic system and liver. His liver had been disturbed for most of his life, due to the biochemical stresses put upon it. Due to his exhaustion over many years, the energy flowing through David's chakras was diminished and his chakras seemed undersized for his emotional and mental development.

My esoteric healing sessions focused on restoring his chakras to a more normal size; restoring energies in his liver, which had been over-burdened with toxic waste; cleansing the lymphatic system, and visualizing particular triangles to balance the nervous system. (Some of these techniques are described in part 2.) David's nerves had been stressed for some years, and I often find, in such cases, that the etheric web that should protect the energy body is damaged. This is one reason that the nervous system can overreact to every stimuli. David often twitched and his muscles jumped during the first healing sessions as a result of the holes in his etheric web.

During David's first visit, I gave him one gram of vitamin C to be taken twice daily; the colloidal mineral salts calcium phosphate and magnesium phosphate for his nerves, repair of ankle bones, and for the panic attacks; the colloidal mineral salts potassium chloride and iron phosphate for the recurrent boils; homeopathic drops for cleansing and toning liver and lymphatic system; and valerian capsules for taking before bed for ease in sleeping. I gave him a homeopathic preparation in a very dilute form, to antidote some of the toxins he had accumulated from chemicals and food. This synthesis of remedies was fairly conservative, as I did not wish to stir up all the toxins too much. David also changed his diet to include more whole foods and raw juices.

After two months on this regimen, David looked much better and his body started to respond by producing severe rashes at times. You will remember how, previously in this chapter, I explained that, in retracing back to health, the acute disease is the first stage, and that skin rashes of various kinds, therefore, often manifest in this stage as the toxins come to the surface. His boils continued. I maintained the basic treatment and added echinacea and cat's claw. I continued his esoteric treatment, with a focus on cleansing the lymphatic system and balancing the nervous system. However, the energy disturbances underlying the areas mentioned were no longer apparent.

After four months of treatment, I introduced another remedy that releases hydrogen and oxygen into the cells. David then had a minor healing crisis in response that included flulike symptoms. He was still suffering from boils, but they appeared less often, and his memory and concentration had improved. Family members were amazed at how improved he seemed. It was of interest to me that when he went off the remedies for two weeks his symptoms started to return. He still suffered headaches, but they were lessening, and so were his dizzy spells. Exposure to photocopying caused him to have a bad attack of dizziness, indicating that his allergies were still a problem. A new carpet in the house caused him to have twitching, another example of his extreme sensitivity to chemicals in the environment.

At this stage, I decided to augment his nerve treatment and added magnesium orotate at 400 mg, twice daily. I changed his herbal mixture to include clivers, red clover, burdock, catmint, and dandelion; this change was to work on his lymphatic system more aggressively. The incidence of boils had diminished, but they still appeared, so I reasoned that they were probably a staphylococcal infection and, accordingly, prescribed this organism, in homeopathic form, to remove the infection. After a few weeks on this remedy, David had no further boils.

Over the next months, David gradually improved in all respects. For a while he worked in New South Wales on a farm and thoroughly enjoyed his outdoor activities. His memory, concentration, and nerves all improved, and he rarely got headaches. His iris now shows a great lessening of toxins in the body. He rarely has skin rashes anymore, and is able to walk through busy streets with far fewer allergy problems than before. For an alternative opinion on his progress, he consulted a therapist who had previously checked his allergies. This therapist found a lessening of David's allergies to wheat, yeast, and pollens, and he noted a lessening of David's allergic response to gasoline fumes.

After David had undergone two years of treatment, I started to taper off the minerals, though he will probably always choose to have health maintenance with a few items, like the antioxidant vitamins C and E, and magnesium for his nerves.

The main reason for including this case is to indicate how a person can retrace back from a very chronic and toxic state to good health. David often comments now how he has to get used to the experience of feeling well, because he felt ill for so many years.

Detoxification by Diet

The average client needs about six months of treatment to increase vitality and reduce toxins. The first few months of treatment include a process called detoxification, which means that the toxins that have accumulated over the years are eliminated through any of the normal channels, such as bowels, kidneys, lungs, or skin. Clients often observe that they get a lot of pimples during this period or have increased mucus in the nose, chest, or on rare occasions, the bowel. It is helpful for a client to help the detoxification period with additions or changes to their diet. This will speed up the process of treating with herbs, minerals, and homeopathics, and the client usually experiences an increase of energy and well-being a few weeks or months after changing their diet.

In fact, our daily vitality and energy are dependent on our diet, as raw foods such as salads and fruits and wholegrain cereals provide most of the subtle energies for our etheric body. Hence, the daily diet is important, not only for detoxifying, but also for building up our physical energies from the life energies present in whole foods, particularly in their uncooked state. Raw foods are very useful for cleansing and detoxification, due to their high enzyme contents; enzymes can be destroyed in normal cooking.

During the detoxifying period, I often direct clients to buy a juice extractor and have at least two glasses daily of freshly made carrot, apple, and celery juice in equal parts, and a lesser amount of beet juice, all preferably from organic produce. When celery is out of season, use the outside leaves of organically grown lettuce. Green beans also make a good green addition, if no green leafy vegetables are available. Make the juice freshly each time you drink it to prevent oxidation. Include the apple to make the juice a bit sweeter and to please the palate; it can be excluded, if you wish.

Other suitable juices include watermelon or pineapple, which give a lovely smooth drink, but not everyone can tolerate pineapple. If people suffer from dysbiosis (disturbed flora of the gut from *Candida albicans*), then using concentrated fruit juice, whether freshly made or bottled, is not a good idea, because the infecting organisms thrive on the sugar. Vegetable juices are preferable in such cases.

The vegetable ingredients of the juices are very alkaline in their effect on the body, and this helps to get rid of acid waste in the tissues. Most people tend to build up acids of various kinds in their tissues from poor nutrition or stress, or both. The blood itself has an in-built alkaline/acid balance, and only becomes imbalanced in severe conditions, like untreated diabetes or chronic renal failure. Generally, the blood off-loads the acid from incorrect diet or stress into the tissues; from a naturopathic viewpoint, this is the basis for much of the tiredness, stiffness, and arthritis experienced in middle and old age.

Apart from the juices, we need to gradually change our daily diet so that once a degree of detoxification has been achieved with juices and naturopathic remedies, our daily diet can do the job without remedies or juices. To do this, include fresh vegetables and salad each day in your diet, and eat at least three pieces of ripe fruit each day, according to whatever is in season. Foods made from white sugar and flour, if taken to excess, add to the acid overload in your tissues. Such foods include most cakes, biscuits, sweets, and chocolates. Meats and cheeses are also acid-forming. The important issue is to have the acid-forming foods in balance with the alkaline vegetables, fruits, and juices. (See appendix 3 for a basic diet sheet written for my clients, used with only minor changes for decades.)

My advice is to start the day with fruit, to "wake up" the digestive enzymes, then have a whole grain cereal with soymilk if there is a need to eliminate dairy products. Midmorning, if you are hungry, have fruit and a handful of almonds or other unsalted nuts (not peanuts because they are subject to the development of potent toxins). For lunch, have a large salad with cottage or feta cheese, tuna, salmon, or lean cold meat, and whole meal or rye bread; or have a salad or roll with the fillings just mentioned. In midafternoon, have fruit or a wholemeal cracker, and for dinner, have at least three vegetables with meat, fish, tofu, eggs, or beans.

Drink lots of water, at least eight glasses per day on an empty stomach. Herbal teas can replace some of this water; even green and black tea will do, keeping in mind that some green teas are high in caffeine. Also, many herbal teas, and certainly ordinary tea, are diuretics (meaning they will increase your urination), so additional water should always be included during your day's water regimen. Limit coffee to one cup daily, and in cases of migraine or severe congestion of the liver, consume no coffee.

Our daily diet is tremendously important, in terms of toxicity and energy levels. But we must also consider the inner factors. This is why I have explained the psychological attributes of the chakras. In terms of our *desire* for certain foods and drinks, we must recall, in particular, the expression of the solar plexus and sacral chakras and their relationship to desire and comfort. People often indulge in "junk" food or drink for emotional comfort. I invariably find that, in cases of obesity and sugar or chocolate craving, these two chakras are disturbed, particularly the sacral center, as it has food, sex, and comfort high on its agenda. No doubt, this is why so many people indulge in junk food for their comfort value.

Remember also that the pancreas is the main endocrine expression of the solar plexus, and it is related to sugar balance in the body through its secretion of insulin. Each time a person craves sugar, there is a rush of energy through the solar plexus to the pancreas and a production of insulin. Over time, this causes a tendency to hypoglycemia or low blood sugar, and the person then craves more sugar, chocolate, or carbohydrates to raise the blood sugar level. But these kinds of foods then cause a sudden drop in blood sugar, due to the insulin surge, and account for the hypoglycemic symptoms. Thus the blood sugar levels go up and down all the time. Eventually, the pancreas becomes tired, and if there is a predisposition in the person's family, diabetes will occur when there is insufficient insulin to deal with excess carbohydrate intake.

This mechanism implies that the real cause and cure of a toxic system must, to some extent, require a redirection of energy on the part of the person who is craving the wrong foods. I see this very plainly in the attitudes of individuals coming for treatment. One will immediately change their diet as soon as I explain the mechanism for the accumulation of waste through eating junk food. Others have a more difficult time because, although they intellectually know the problems of junk food, they cannot seem to control their lower chakras. This is where meditation and esoteric healing can be a great help, but even then a certain amount of willpower has to be exerted by the client.

It takes months, and sometimes years, to correct accumulated toxins. Usually, the first improvement after holistic treatment with natural therapies begins with an increase of energy, and this improvement in vitality often starts the process of elimination through bowel, kidneys, lungs, and skin. This is usually a gradual process, with no particular side effects, but occasionally there is liver discomfort, diarrhea, abdominal pain, and excessive mucus production. In these cases, the treatment can be slowed down if the patient feels ill, although some clients like to get their health restored as quickly as possible, despite discomfort for a few days or weeks.

When the body eliminates waste very quickly after a boost in vitality, the process is called a healing crisis. The healing crisis can include symptoms of headaches, diarrhea, liver discomfort, and elimination of mucus from chest, throat, nose, and bowel. More commonly, individuals get slowly better with improved energy and gradual elimination of their symptoms.

We can consider the healing crisis and the disease crisis in the form of two simple equations. The healing crisis can be represented by the equation: *vitality + toxins → a healing crisis with elimination of waste.* In other words, if the person has reasonable vitality and you increase it further with holistic treatment, they will start to eliminate the toxins, either dramatically or gradually, depending on the level of vitality. On the other hand, if their vitality is diminishing and toxins are increasing, we will have another equation: *low vitality + toxins → disease crisis and possibly death.* This means that the organs gradually become diseased, and chronic disease of various kinds gradually moves the individual in the direction of death.

The Circle of Disease Involving Vitality and Toxins

We can regard the etheric body as the seat of our body energies or vitality. Diminished etheric energies lead to an accumulation of toxins as each cell in each tissue eliminates less waste due to increasingly sluggish function. On the other hand, if the body becomes toxic due to poor diet and an overload of chemicals from various sources in food, our environment, or pharmaceutical drugs, the vitality will greatly diminish. So the end result is the same: poor energy and toxic overload. We thus have a vicious circle, and it is the task of the therapist to work out what comes first, poor lifestyle, resulting in less energy and the consequent accumulation of toxins or accumulation of toxins, resulting in lowered energies in the etheric body.

Our vitality diminishes and the level of toxins develops as a gradual process over the years, roughly in the stages of acute, subacute, and chronic, as discussed earlier in this chapter.

Summary: The two aims of naturopathic practice are to build up vitality and remove toxins. Vitality is intimately related to the etheric body and its health. Iris diagnosis is a handy tool to get an overview of the level of vitality and amount of toxins in the body. The clear iris of the newborn indicates how we start life with a clean slate, and we see from the iris how toxins accumulate over the years and how vitality diminishes.

Vitality is also related to the capacity for inner alignment. The esoteric healing described in the cases already mentioned allows for energies to flow into the body, improving general well-being and vitality. So vitality can be enhanced by using physical remedies to remove toxins and build up the physical nervous system, and also by bringing in subtle energies to restore the energies *underlying* our organs and tissues.

Natural therapists see the three stages of disease as related to diminishing energy and accumulating toxins, rather than as the activity of infectious organisms. Acute, sub-acute, and chronic diseases are, therefore, viewed by natural therapists in a different way than by orthodox medical practitioners. Chronic diseases are viewed as connected to a gradual accumulation of toxins, and they are not seen as isolated from the earlier acute and sub-acute stages of disease. Thus, the naturopath views bacteria or viruses, on their own, as a serious threat only when our system is severely out of balance. The naturopathic experience finds that during holistic treatment, an individual will ideally retrace back through the various stages from chronic to acute manifestations.

The healing and disease crises are described by two simple equations:

Vitality + toxins → *a healing crisis with elimination of waste.* Certain discomfort may be experienced during the healing crisis but vitality generally increases, despite increased elimination through the normal channels of bowel, kidneys, lung, and skin.

Low vitality + toxins → *disease crisis and possibly death.* In this case, the accumulation of toxins finally over-burdens body organs and various serious conditions, such as severe arthritis or cancer, or serious nervous problems, such as multiple sclerosis, can develop. The cycle of disease can start at either end—poor vitality or toxic overload.

Good nutrition and suitable diets are cornerstones of naturopathic treatment, and are part of the detoxification process and essential for the building of vitality. Clients are trained to use raw juices and foods for cleansing, and to concentrate on whole foods.

In part 2, we will look at specific categories of disease and examine many case histories, for which I outline both the natural therapies and the esoteric healing treatment. I am not going to include every possible disease, but I will explore disorders in connection with energy disturbances of the chakras that affect a large number of people. Hence, we will explore issues like immunity, respiratory problems, reproductive disorders, and nervous problems along with the related chakra. This will underscore the need to understand holistic treatment as a *synthesis* of physical remedies and esoteric healing.

PART TWO

Introduction

This is the practical part, where I describe case histories illustrating how the natural medicines in each case are blended successfully with esoteric healing for optimal healing. To help establish the links between the chakras and various diseases, the cases are divided into sections that relate to each chakra. For instance, the solar plexus will be linked with the digestive system, lymphatic problems will go with the throat chakra, and reproductive problems with the sacral chakra.

After each chapter, there are exercises to balance the chakra concerned and to apply the associated triangles. In appendix 1, you will find a spreadsheet for all the triangles and a review of all the exercises, in relation to each chakra and body system.

You need to remember that energy follows thought, so it is wise to proceed slowly and gently if you intend to use these triangles on relatives and friends. The exercises given will be found to be very rewarding, and can also be used on your pet animals. Read the sections of ailments connected to each chakra in part two *before* starting to practice the triangles. This will give you the necessary understanding so that the exercises can be used for best effect.

Each chapter in part 2 starts with a brief review of points about the chakra involved and its related organs and tissues, and has a discussion of the associated medical problems and their naturopathic, and its esoteric explanation. The case histories offer a brief medical history of each person, including their physical ailment, my diagnosis, both exoteric and esoteric, the naturopathic and esoteric treatment, and a summary of the outcome.

There may seem to be more emphasis in some sections than others because, in the average person, there is more emphasis on one chakra than the others. For instance, the solar plexus chakra is associated with emotional upsets and governs, therefore, nearly all digestive disturbances. Because the average person is emotionally focused, a large percentage of individuals are subject to digestive disorders. Humanity is also very intelligent and creative, and this emphasizes the throat chakra, lymphatic problems and, therefore, many infections. Due to the awakening heart center within humanity, heart and circulatory disorders are also prominent, as are many immune problems, due to the relationship between the thymus gland and the heart.

I have been pleased to find, over the last few years, that esoteric healing gives the physical remedies a good "kick start," and that the various disorders seem to resolve much more quickly as a result of this synthesis in practice. This is because, unless the energy field is corrected, the use of the natural medicines alone will not correct the problems in the energy field.

I have been pleased to find, over the last few years, that esoteric healing gives the physical remedies a good "kick start," and that the various disorders seem to resolve much more quickly as a result of this synthesis in practice. This is because, unless the energy field is corrected, the use of the natural medicines alone will not correct the problems in the energy field. There will sometimes be a dramatic improvement in the condition without esoteric healing, but if the energy field is not corrected, the disorder may later relapse when the person tapers off their remedies.

I usually see my clients only once per month, except for acute cases. When I first added this modality of subtle healing to my practice and was able to correct the energy disturbances, I expected that, after a month, the energy field could have relapsed. To my delight, I have found that, except in cases like advanced cancer or profound psychological disturbance, the etheric field of most clients has remained balanced after treatment. Occasionally, for an individual subject to electromagnetic disturbance, such as sleeping on an electric blanket or sitting for long periods under fluorescent lights, there may be recurring energy field disturbances.

The aim of esoteric healing, as stated in chapter 5, is to contact our healing essence, the soul.[33] Obviously, not all my clients are interested to undertake a regular practice of meditation that might continue their soul alignments between the monthly visits or after the treatment is tapered off. I find that clients vary greatly as to how they respond to the healing. Most experience peace and serenity; a few see colors; a few others have visions of various kinds. At the time of the healing, there is a flow of energy from the soul of the healer to the soul of the client, and the healing will take place whether the client has any psychic or spiritual experience or not. Their overall experience is relaxation and peace.

Although the subtle healing underpins the physical remedies, the healing without the natural medicines may not be completely successful, because there are often profound deficiencies and physiological disturbances in the clients. It is the *synthesis* of the healing and natural medicines that seems to create total healing.

Although I have tried to keep a logical sequence to the case histories, there is a lot of interaction between the various chakras, and even from a medical viewpoint, between various bodily systems for each ailment. I will discuss the chakras and associated problems in the order that has been taught in esoteric healing courses for the last 25 years.

Therefore, we will start with the solar plexus chakra and its associated digestive problems. The reason for starting here, rather than moving in sequence down or up the spine, is because the solar plexus relates to our emotions, which profoundly affect our physical health. I have found that if this chakra is balanced early in the process, the healing is more effective later.

We can then track the various ailments associated with each chakra in the order that we balance the chakras (after balancing the solar plexus). That order is base chakra, sacral chakra, heart chakra, throat chakra, and brow chakra.

7 The Solar Plexus and Gastrointestinal Challenges

We start our journey through the practical sequence of ailments with the solar plexus. This is the first chakra to be balanced when learning the esoteric healing protocol, partly due to our emotional focus via this center, and partly because, in naturopathic philosophy, most disease is said to start in the digestive system, which is conditioned by the solar plexus.

The solar plexus chakra expresses all our desires, including our desire for food, and this is the basis for many health problems if our choice of food is inappropriate. Another important consideration in connection with the solar plexus relates to the effect of negative emotions on our digestive functions. If energy flows harmoniously through this chakra, our digestion is usually good, even if our diet is not very well-balanced.

As the solar plexus conditions all our digestive functions, so its energy relates to the pancreas, stomach, liver, gallbladder, small intestine, and the first three-quarters of the large intestine. The digestive disorders conditioned by our solar plexus energy include diarrhea, constipation, gallstones, liver problems like hepatitis, intestinal candidiasis, diabetes, and cancer of some part of the digestive tract.

The endocrine gland associated with this chakra is the pancreas, which produces insulin to keep us supplied with an even amount of energy, derived from carbohydrates. The pancreas also produces pancreatic "juice" for the purpose of digesting carbohydrates, proteins, and fats. We will explore the inner and outer causes in the area of digestive disturbances.

Digestive disturbances feature very strongly in my clinical practice. Many of these problems stem from inappropriate diet, although, generally, people are much better educated about diet than thirty years ago, when I first started to practice natural therapies. The public has been exposed to a media explosion of interest in health, fitness, and eating well, and even if individuals are addicted to the wrong types of food, they tend to know what they *should* be eating, even if they don't do it.

In the twenty-first century, a major factor in gastrointestinal problems relates to stress. Whether the problem is heartburn, ulcers, irritable bowel syndrome, diarrhea, or constipation, stress on the nervous system is often a major contributing cause, so we'll consider this first.

The Nervous System and Digestive Problems

A basic nervous imbalance is caused by stress from overwork, lack of sleep, or lack of relaxation. These factors stimulate the sympathetic part of the autonomic nervous system, which is related to the adrenal glands. These glands pour out adrenalin and cortisone, and prepare us for fight-or-flight reactions. At the same time, the parasympathetic system, closely involved with the vagus nerve, is suppressed and digestion thereby suffers.

An outer factor relating to nervous stress may involve nutrient deficiencies. Through stress, we tend to use up the mineral magnesium, a mineral already lacking in our soils, due to poor farming methods. Thus, eating foods high in magnesium, such as dark green leafy vegetables and almonds, may not suffice for our nutrient needs. A lack of magnesium in our body results in all sorts of spasms throughout the gut, and this further inhibits our digestive juices from flowing adequately; it may also lead to pain and inflammation. We could say that magnesium deficiency is part of the outer cause for nervous problems relating to the gastrointestinal tract.[34]

From the inner perspective, the solar plexus chakra is related to all digestive organs. When we are emotionally disturbed, this chakra often goes into spasm or, alternatively, it becomes enlarged and opens too wide. Thus, when we get upset, we sometimes try to shut off from emotional impacts, and this can cause the energy to be withdrawn from the solar plexus chakra, which then appears to be partially shut down, causing spasm, and sometimes pain, just above the navel. This lack of a free flow of energy will, in turn, cause a lack of digestive "juices" from the stomach, liver, and pancreas, which results in weak digestion. The congestion of the gall bladder, resulting from withdrawal, and hence, stasis of energy, may cause gallstones.

Alternatively, in a different type of person who is more emotionally expressive, the energy in the solar plexus may become excessive, and emotional disturbance produces an excess of stomach acid, resulting in stomach ulcers. In this situation the chakra may appear enlarged and too open, compared to the other chakras. Often, people complain of pain around or just above the navel. Pathology evaluations of this area reveal nothing, because the cause of the pain is from the chakra in the etheric body, which underlies the physical body (as described in chapter 3) and not in the abdominal area physically.

The final effect of energy disturbances in the solar plexus is contraction, often in the small or large intestines, such that poor digestion, diarrhea, and constipation may result. This is the chain: *emotional stress → solar plexus cramp → vagus nerve inhibition → bowel cramp → diarrhea or constipation.* If the condition persists for years, then more serious ailments can develop from lack of blood and nerve supply to the area, plus an accompanying accumulation of waste as in constipation. Stomach and duodenal ulcers can result from an imbalance of gastric and pancreatic secretions as part of a disturbance in subtle energy flow. The following case is a typical and fairly straightforward one of weak digestion with both inner and outer causes.

A Case of Weak Digestion: Kylie, 20, visited me for abdominal pain, diarrhea alternating with constipation, nausea, and exhaustion. She had lost seventeen pounds. Her iris indicated a weakness in the mineral status needed for the nervous system; this was revealed by the fact that all the radial iris fibers were slightly wavy and separated, instead of being straight. The bronchial areas, as illustrated in the iris, were weak. Although she did not have much of a build up of toxins, an energy scan indicated that her liver and small and large intestines were disturbed in their function. This case clearly illustrates how the irregular flow of energy through the solar plexus causes diarrhea when there is an excess of energy, and constipation when there is a deficiency of energy.

My naturopathic treatment for Kylie included an herbal mixture of angelica, melissa, red clover, catmint, and centaury. These herbs were to tone and stimulate her digestive organs. To stabilize her nervous system, I gave Kylie the tissue salts potassium and magnesium phosphate, and I prescribed chromium for her sugar craving. Her treatment also included flower essences for emotional balancing, and homeopathic drops for liver and lymphatic toning.

After I conducted the main chakra balancing and vitality triangles, I visualized the digestive triangles. The digestive triangles involve the following triangles between solar plexus, liver, and liver minor; solar plexus, stomach, and stomach minor; and between the organs themselves, liver, stomach, and pancreas. The sacral triangle on Kylie was then visualized to balance her reproductive organs; this one involves a triangle between the sacral center and the ovary minor chakras. In addition, I did the grounding triangles (sacral chakra, sacral center and hip minor chakras, sacral center and knee minors, and sacral center and foot minors). The final technique to regulate her periods was the use of the "endocrine pentagon," which includes a visualization of five points: pituitary gland, two adrenal minor chakras, and two ovarian minor chakras.

The grounding triangles were included because my impression of Kylie was that she was not quite in her body, and this made her vulnerable to infection and viruses. As part of this other-worldliness, Kylie was having trouble knowing what she wanted to do in life and what direction to take as a career. We had some discussions as to the meaning of life, and she was very interested in the esoteric perspective of the healing process. She now belongs to a metaphysical study group, and does regular meditation.

Kylie had about twelve months of successful treatment, but she relapsed whenever she ate junk food. She then went overseas for a few months and had extensive immunizations to prepare for the trip. While away, she suffered a lot of flulike symptoms. She was very exhausted on her return, and had symptoms similar to chronic fatigue syndrome. Another member of her family had also suffered this problem. I found her thymus gland and lymphatic system to be in a disturbed state, and believed this problem was probably responsible for her low immunity.

Further healing on a weekly basis corrected Kylie's thymus gland and immune system problems, and she noticed the healing made a huge improvement in her energy level. It took a few sessions to correct the thymus gland so that it did not relapse. Kylie was then so improved that she was able to get a job. Her treatment has since been tapered off, although she needs to stay on the mineral salts to keep her nervous system in balance.

This seemed a fairly simple case, in which weakness in the nervous system caused most of the digestive and immune problems. Fears also featured at times. Fear of travel was one that beset Kylie before her overseas trip, as well as fear of being separated from her family. Kylie had a type of mystical openness that seemed to interfere with the manifestation of strength needed to function in the outer world. She did not seem to be able to focus clearly on managing or moving her life in a definite direction. These conditions thus needed inner and outer treatment, and, as always, I cannot say that one was more important than the other.

After a few months, Kylie returned for treatments, as she was starting to have mild viral problems. The energy in her thymus gland was again disturbed. I wondered why this problem was repeating and, on questioning her, found she did a long meditation using a mantra twice daily. I wondered if this type of meditation was causing her to become ungrounded, such that there was insufficient energy in the immune system, including the thymus gland. I asked her to think about this situation, because perhaps a rift had developed between her physical and etheric bodies, depleting her of energy, which should be flowing through the immune system. For health and good energy, we need the etheric body to be tightly *connected* to our physical body.

I had the impression that, in keeping with Kylie's perceived vagueness, her energies were generally not flowing right down into the physical body via the etheric body, and perhaps the thymus gland was the weak point affected by this energy depletion. So, in her case, there was possibly a withdrawal or abstraction of energy due to an overly mystical temperament and this was, in turn, depleting the solar plexus (digestion) and heart chakra (thymus gland). In fact, whenever she had bouts of ill health, I found these chakras to be generally depleted.

After another two sessions of healing and the regular use of her supplements, Kylie felt much stronger, and she started a new job with individuals who have suffered brain injuries. She is most suitable for this job, with her gentle and loving nature, and she enjoys this work. After she had been working a couple of months, she was tired, but I was pleased to find from scanning her energy that her chakras remained a normal size and that the thymus was not disturbed.

This case illustrates several points of my thesis. First, it shows the effect of too little and then too much energy through the solar plexus, which conditions the digestion, causing constipation to alternate with diarrhea. Second, it illustrates the interaction between the various chakras such that, apart from the solar plexus disturbance (which recurred due to fear of leaving home to go overseas), there was also a disturbance of energy in the thymus gland that affected her immunity. There is a close connection between the solar plexus and the heart, as they are both concerned with love and relationships.

The third point of interest is that as disturbance can also come from outer causes, it appears that the thymus gland may have not only been disturbed through fears when Kylie went overseas, but also from the extensive round of immunizations she had before she left. The thymus gland relates to the maturation of T lymphocyte cells, and the interaction with other white blood cells to produce antibodies. A person with a sensitive immune system can find it temporarily disturbed following immunizations.

Finally, when Kylie obtained a stimulating job, her energies seemed to be more focused on daily living, and she began to stay consistently healthy. This justifies my suspicion that she was previously ungrounded. Her joy in her job invokes energies to flow into every part of her body, and the soul energies she contacts in her meditation are now used in the outer work she does to help disadvantaged people.

Constipation Case Study: Constipation is probably one of the most common and simple disorders involving our digestive system. It can have interrelated causes that may include poor diet with little roughage and raw foods, a sluggish liver, or sluggish thyroid gland activity. There may be a weakness in the elastic tissue of the intestines or a deficiency of the mineral salts necessary for healthy nerve cell tone.

From an inner perspective, constipation can generally be assumed to be a stasis or blockage of energy, involving the solar plexus and sacral centers. It is of interest that psychologists have spoken about constipation as the inability to let go. This is probably an oversimplification of a situation whereby the energies are not flowing through these two chakras for a number of reasons. As with most conditions, the therapist must decide whether the inner or outer factors (described in the previous paragraph) need the most attention, as was the situation in the next case history.

Anna visited me for constipation, saying her intestines only "worked" every four days. She had pain in the right groin area that was likely caused by a buildup of feces near the ileocecal valve, located near the appendix. A laparoscopy had revealed no abnormalities. Her iris was fairly clear, but the observable fibers were slightly wavy, indicating a lack of the basic minerals needed for the nervous system.

Her first prescription included a digestive mixture containing motherwort, dandelion, centaury, burdock, red clover; homeopathic drops for liver and lymphatic toning; and colloidal and potassium phosphate for nerve balancing. Basic esoteric healing techniques were used to balance her chakras and, for this, I included the digestive triangles (see as in the previous case). On her return visit, Anna reported that she had moved her bowels every day and that the pain in her right side had gone.

This was an interesting contrast to the previous case with Kylie, as Anna responded in just one month. Such a result indicates to me that there were no deep energy blocks of any kind. Indeed, when I did the healing, I did not find any major problems with the chakras, in terms of imbalance. The healing seemed to give the remedies an added push to restore homeostasis in the body.

Sometimes there is a general weakness of the digestion that results from lowered vitality or from a poor connection between the energy field (etheric body) and the physical body. Weak digestion can also result from mineral deficiencies. In many cases of digestive ailments, the diet has played a major part in the evolution of the problem. For instance, the continual eating of junk food and fast food can be a major contributing factor to problems with the liver, gallbladder, and intestines. The next case involves poor diet and a consequent vulnerability to infectious organisms often found in food, especially prepared fast foods.

Irritable Bowel Syndrome Case Study: Of the many cases of this syndrome I've seen, I usually find a combination of inflammation, consequent spasm, and poor digestive capacity involved. This condition can have many causes, including poor diet, viruses, bacteria, and use of prescription drugs. Such problems can go on for years, yet they usually resolve when the digestive system is toned up with a few herbs and an appropriate type of magnesium for muscle spasms. Clients with this complaint have usually been in need of magnesium for some time, and there may be other signs for this mineral, such as tension headaches.

Jenny needed help with irritable bowel syndrome, diagnosed two years before after a bout of salmonella poisoning. She suffered flatulence, bloating, and abdominal discomfort. She had a history of mouth ulcers, and her diet was not good, featuring white bread, lots of coffee, and canned fruits. My energy scan indicated energy disturbances in the liver and the small and large intestines.

Naturopathic treatment included a digestive mixture of dandelion, centaury, meadowsweet, red clover, and a tiny amount of goldenseal. I also gave Jenny acidophilus, bifidus, and bulgaris cultures in a capsule to restore her intestinal flora, plus magnesium orotate for bowel spasm, and homeopathic liver and lymph toning drops.

The original salmonella infection could be considered as a big shock to the system, and I find that even months, and sometimes years, after such an assault on the body, shock can still be present. Such shock affects the various parts of the autonomic nervous system and, as this system is not under the control of the will, the digestive system can be considerably affected. It is necessary to stimulate the vagus nerve via the vagus triangle.

My session of esoteric healing, after the basic chakra balancing, included the digestive triangles, lymphatic drainage, shock triangle (solar plexus minor, ileocecal valve, and descending colon) for the original salmonella infection, and the vagus triangle to rebalance her nervous system. This latter triangle is of particular importance in balancing the autonomic system in digestive disorders. This treatment results in restoring the balance between the vagus nerve (parasympathetic nervous system) and the overactive sympathetic part of the nervous system. The vagus triangle consists of the brow center, the vagus minor chakra, situated above the heart, and another important minor center, the alta major chakra in the back of the neck, situated where the spine joins the skull (see chapter 4 for a description).

On her return visit after a month, Jenny reported more energy and considerable improvement in her intestines. She had improved her diet by cutting out white bread and including more fresh fruit. At further visits, she mentioned there was some relapse whenever she got stressed at work or missed taking her remedies. Ideally, she should have been having weekly healing instead of monthly, but she is now in a stable condition after staying on minimum naturopathic treatment for fifteen months.

Jenny's case is a good one to illustrate both inner and outer factors affecting her health. She mentioned herself how stress at work affects her digestion, and this is the inner factor that conditions the energies flowing through her solar plexus chakra. Another inner factor relates to her regular relapses from a good diet and her desire for junk food at times. Our desires get expressed through the solar plexus chakra, as mentioned earlier. During the treatment time, she has become much more aware of these dietary factors and the fact that natural medicines can help her through times of stress and poor diet. When she becomes free from stress and maintains a good diet on a long-term basis, she will need few physical remedies. This case shows how the synthesis of outer and inner treatment helped her system regain balance.

Food Sensitivities and Allergies

Some individuals move from a condition in which there is a moderate problem with poor diet, weak digestion, and subsequent discomfort, to a more extreme state of food sensitivities and allergies. Nothing makes my heart sink faster than when a client arrives for the first appointment with a big bag of remedies given to them by a succession of natural therapists. She will then proceed to explain that her digestion is "terrible," and how she can tolerate only a few foods and that even these are starting to give her problems. More often than not, these clients are underweight and seem to be obsessed with their health.

In considering the esoteric causes of disease, I find that it is essential for such clients to lift the focus of their attention off the point of friction. The "point of friction" is an Alice Bailey term, found under what she called the Fourth Law of Healing: the individual exacerbates or worsens their disease by constantly focusing their thoughts and emotions on the disease. The constant worrying creates friction in the area of concern. If the therapist can help the client to align with their inner essence, especially through the practice of meditation, healing energies can flow to the trouble spot and relieve the friction.

This is easier said than done, and these individuals are often classic therapy-resistant patients. The more they think about every twinge, cramp, and bloat, the more enhanced it all seems to become. They are often very intelligent, but unless they can find another focus for their intelligence apart from their digestion, it is almost impossible to treat them successfully. In such cases, the solar plexus is usually found to be imbalanced and can be either too large or too small, compared with the other chakras; there are usually also chaotic energy patterns in most of the digestive organs.

I mention these extreme cases to make the point of mind-body interaction; that is, to show the effect of disturbed emotions and thoughts on the body. In less extreme cases, the same principle applies to a lesser degree. There can be many causes of weak digestion, but, in general, we need to maintain a semblance of serenity and reasonable eating habits for good digestion. Even moderate excitement can inhibit the digestive juices via the sympathetic nervous system, so it is not a good idea, for example, to habitually watch your favorite police drama while eating.

Individuals can develop sensitivities to certain foods through slight imbalances in the immune system that increase levels of particular antibodies. The proliferation of these antibodies when we eat these foods is accompanied by inflammation and swelling of the mucous membrane in the small and large bowel. However, in light of my previous comments about the interaction of mind and emotions on the body, it is hard to know which comes first—the chicken or the egg. Researchers have discovered that changes in the immune system happen within minutes of changes in our emotional states, so it is possible that many of our food sensitivities are related to factors in our psyche.

Somewhat related to modern immunological findings about food allergies is the concept from anthroposophical medicine, as pioneered by Rudolf Steiner. He suggests that we need a strong digestion to de-nature our food, meaning, to overcome something that is essentially foreign to our body.[35] So even before science discovered reactive antibodies, Steiner reasoned that some people with a lack of etheric energy in the digestive system are unable to cope with certain foods, because the food acts as a foreign body. This scenario is very close to the modern findings, whereby irritable bowel syndrome is understood to result from antibodies secreted in response to certain foods.

We should also consider the possible effect from fluoridation of water supplies in relation to the strength of our digestive enzymes and food sensitivities. Biochemists used fluoride as an enzyme poison in almost the same strengths as it is placed in water supplies—one part fluoride per one million parts of water. Consider the possible effect on our digestive enzymes if we drink the recommended eight glasses of (tap) water daily, or the effect on a child's digestion if they swallow fluoridated toothpaste that is usually many thousands times that strength in fluoride content. It may be a coincidence, but I noticed a large increase of irritable bowel syndrome a few years after Australian drinking water was fluoridated.

It appears that we need healthy digestive enzymes to adequately deal with our foods, and that these enzymes can be enhanced by raw foods and juices and may possibly be affected by both our emotional states and by additives such as fluoride. A poor diet of refined foods, plus foods containing many chemicals, may also effect the largest metabolic factory in the body—the liver.

Liver Problems

I have described two examples of simple digestive problems resulting from poor diet and/or nervous stress, and have shown the effect of the mind on the digestion via the autonomic nervous system. We can now begin to consider more serious digestive ailments involving organic changes or pathology, starting with the liver. The liver is our major organ for metabolism and has many roles, including the production of bile, which assists in the absorption of fats. The liver also produces antibodies to fight disease, and it is involved with the production of glycogen (sugar) and an important protein called albumin.

One important daily activity of the liver is detoxification of drugs and chemicals taken into the body. You can appreciate the burden put on our livers in our polluted culture. Chemicals are added to our water, industrial pollutants contaminate our air, thousands of chemicals are in our food, multiple pharmaceutical drugs are prescribed by the medical profession, and chemicals are absorbed via our cosmetics. Toxic substances the liver cannot detoxify frequently accumulate in the lymphatic system, so it's no wonder natural therapists treat nearly everyone with detoxification medicines for the liver and lymph system, regardless of the ailment patients present.

In addition to congestion caused in the liver by an overload of chemicals, there are liver infections from several types of viruses, causing hepatitis or inflammation of the liver. Permanent liver problems can originate from hepatitis types B and C; immunization is available against hepatitis B, but not against C. Both viral strains can cause permanent damage in the form of cirrhosis, scarring of the liver, and even liver cancer.[36]

Hepatitis C is considered to be a silent epidemic, a time bomb waiting to go off, because it is only the last few years that blood donations were screened for this virus. This means that many people having surgery or treatment for injuries may have received blood containing the hepatitis C virus. This virus often has no symptoms for many years and, therefore, at this point in time, the extent of its spread is unknown. After some years, the person with latent hepatitis C can develop liver problems, such as cirrhosis, that greatly impede liver function.

You may ask how, in the case of hepatitis, the associated chakra—solar plexus—is affected. In the next case, this relationship is shown, as the subject contracted his hepatitis C through taking drugs intravenously. Any addiction is related to the desires of the solar plexus for particular sensations. In addition, it is chiefly as a result of drug addicts infecting blood supplies that the virus has caused this community health problem. Both hepatitis B and C are contracted from an infected person through blood contact, as in dirty syringes, blood transfusions, or from other body fluids such as saliva.

Hepatitis Case Study: John, 35, had hepatitis C. He came to me for help with his gallstones, but on taking his history, I found his case was complicated by the fact that he had contracted hepatitis C from dirty syringe use when he took intravenous drugs as a young man. He was on a disability pension following a car accident, and had a very poor lifestyle in terms of diet and activities. His diet included a lot of ham and cheese sandwiches, plus lots of coffee. No wonder his liver was disturbed, apart from the hepatitis; this diet itself is a challenge to the liver.

John smoked and drank a lot of beer, and he usually went to sleep from four A.M. onwards, after watching hours of television, and then slept most of the morning. In this case, his liver and gallbladder function was complicated by the hepatitis virus. If the liver is not functioning well, gallstones are easily formed due to sluggish bile activity.

John's self-esteem was very poor, and he was overweight and exhausted. When he first visited me three years ago, he had sharp pains in the gallbladder area and was trying to find a way to avoid having his gallbladder removed. The presence of gallbladder stones had shown up in an ultrasound test. His iris indicated a moderate degree of toxins throughout the gastrointestinal tract, and it had mild nerve rings, which show as white rings in the iris. On scanning his energy field, I found the disturbance in the liver and gallbladder showed up strongly as a chaotic pattern of energies.

When I first started the synthesis in healing approach, I always felt a bit reticent about suggesting esoteric healing to men who had no obvious esoteric interests. However, I soon found that they loved the quiet time of relaxation. John was no exception, and he sometimes saw colors behind his closed eyes during the healing sessions. So I was mistaken in thinking that only women would be sensitive to the inner energies contacted.

I gave John directions about his diet, to encourage him to cut out cheese and to have more whole foods, including fresh salads and fruit. For his gallbladder, I gave him tinctures of chelidonium and turmeric (fifteen drops before meals), plus an herbal tablet with St. Mary's thistle and dandelion for his liver function. Clinical trials with St. Mary's thistle have shown that it protects the membranes of liver cells from free radical activity and promotes regeneration of the liver through stimulating the production of hepatocytes.[37] I gave John vitamin C (1 g, twice daily) for detoxification and to counteract his smoking, vitamin B complex to raise his energy level, and I included my usual liver and lymphatic homeopathic drops.

After one month, John reported that he had changed his diet in a positive way and that he had more energy. He was walking daily and, most importantly, the sharp pains in his gallbladder had ceased. We had a talk about his sleeping habits and I advised him to gradually go to bed earlier each week until he was able to go to sleep before midnight. His treatment was continued for many months and included the esoteric healing aspects.

His healing, apart from the main chakra balancing, included the digestive triangles (because the liver and gallbladder were involved), plus the clearing triangle, to help eliminate old emotional issues. (This latter triangle involves the brow chakra, heart, and solar plexus, and is described in detail in chapter 14.) After some months, when he was looking to move out into the working world, the "triangle of becoming" was included in his program; this one involves the crown, heart, and base chakras.

He gradually returned to a normal sleeping pattern and reduced his smoking and drinking. Sometimes he would eat the wrong foods and his gallbladder would play up again. After some months, we started to talk about what he would like to do in his life, and he began to think in terms of creative activities. John started to do part-time work. He had a temporary setback with relatives staying in the house who made him feel very irritable, but he recovered when they left. The liver and gallbladder are the main focus for anger and irritation, especially if their expression is suppressed, so whenever John gets upset, his gallbladder plays up.

He is now talking about retraining for more permanent work, and his self-esteem has improved greatly. Even if he eventually needs to have the gallbladder removed, his body and overall being are in a much better condition to have the surgery and to recuperate. His hepatitis C will also be greatly improved by the general treatment he is taking.

In summary, the physical and esoteric medicine worked together to place John in a completely different space. He is working part time, and is finding that he can cope with difficult personal relations much better. I have taught him simple meditation and visualization techniques that he has used to control his anger. This is good, as the liver and gallbladder are often called the seat of the emotions and are related to anger in Chinese medicine. John now rarely has any gallbladder discomfort and, apart from the physical causes for his liver congestion due to poor diet and heavy drinking in the past, learning to control his anger has been a big factor in his improvement. The esoteric healing helped keep his solar plexus chakra balanced, a necessary step, as this chakra is related to all emotions, including anger. Lately, he has mentioned how much his motivation has increased and that he is mentally much improved.

Gallstones Case Study: Mark's gallbladder case had no accompanying liver damage. He wished to avoid surgery and was referred to me by a medical doctor. He is a 45-year-old nursing and naturopathic lecturer who had suffered an attack of severe pain prior to visiting me. An ultrasound revealed that multiple gallstones had triggered his pain. Mark is a vegetarian with a fairly good diet. An etheric scan revealed disturbance of the liver and gallbladder and of his solar plexus chakra.

I gave Mark homeopathic drops for the liver and gallbladder, the same gallbladder drops as in John's case, the herbs chelidonium and turmeric, and magnesium phosphate for spasm of the gallbladder and bile duct; this was combined with homeopathic iron phosphate for inflammation of the gallbladder. I added vitamin B complex later for energy and the Bach flower essences Mimulus, Cherry Plum, Impatiens, Vervain, and Cerato for stress, fear, and for building confidence.

The esoteric healing involved chakra balancing plus the digestive triangles, including the gallbladder triangle. The adrenal triangle—base chakra and the two adrenal minor chakras (see appendix 1)—was added for stress, as Mark had a lot of work challenges in his lecturing job at a local university. His temperament is in complete contrast to the previous case, as he pushes himself hard in his work and is a high achiever who probably needs to slack off. In the last case, the opposite situation prevailed, where John needed to be motivated to work at all. In both cases, strong emotions via the solar plexus were involved, but the anger, in Mark's case, was different, and much more controlled and suppressed. There were also personal challenges, and during the course of treatment, he decided to separate from his partner, after which a lot of conflict disappeared from his life.

Mark found after a few weeks of treatment that he was able to eat foods that previously upset his gallbladder and that he rarely suffered further pain. He continues the treatment with monthly visits and is pleased with his steady improvement. Occasionally, he has a relapse if he overworks, in which case, he has an emergency remedy of high potency homeopathic Berberis. He has had to use his remedy, plus extra magnesium phosphate tablets, on only a few occasions.

Gallstones are not likely to disappear quickly with either natural medicines or subtle healing. The gallbladder has an important function in concentrating the bile for the purpose of fat digestion, and if the gallbladder itself can be kept healthy, it is preferable not to have it removed. Keeping stable solar plexus energy and learning to deal with anger and stress are of particular importance for the liver and gallbladder. Therefore, a *synthesis* of natural medicines and esoteric work can deal with both the inner and outer factors conditioning the function of liver and gallbladder.

Diabetes

We now move to diabetes, a very common disorder that is increasing in incidence in Western countries. It is closely related to the solar plexus chakra and its material expression, the endocrine gland called the pancreas. The solar plexus conditions all our digestive organs, but, in particular, the pancreas, which has an endocrine secretion of insulin and an exocrine digestive fluid of pancreatic juice. This digestive juice has enzymes that deal with three of our major food categories, namely, carbohydrates, fats, and proteins. From a naturopathic viewpoint, the pancreas is often deficient in its secretion of pancreatic juice long before diabetes occurs. This means that the pancreatic juice in such cases is deficient in enzymes that help digest carbohydrates, fats, and proteins. Diabetes occurs when the pancreas can no longer cope properly in managing carbohydrate metabolism.

Diabetes is of two kinds: insulin dependent diabetes (Type 1) and noninsulin dependent diabetes (Type 2). This second kind usually occurs from middle age onwards and is often associated with obesity. There is often a family tendency to the disease but, given the explosion of diabetes over the last few decades, this is obviously not always the case.[38]

> *Keeping stable solar plexus energy and learning to deal with anger and stress are of particular importance for the liver and gallbladder. Therefore, a synthesis of natural medicines and esoteric work can deal with both the inner and outer factors conditioning the function of liver and gallbladder.*

121

Diabetes, especially Type 2, is, in many ways, a disease directly expressing disturbed solar plexus activity. Type 2 diabetes does not include the early destruction of pancreatic cells that takes place as in Type 1 diabetes. Some Type 2 diabetics are known to have an inherited predisposition to this disorder, but the majority of persons suffering Type 2 diabetes are overweight. This fact correlates with my understanding that the solar plexus chakra conditions desires, including desires for food, and, often, for too much food.

Continual eating of excess sweets over many years can eventually cause insulin resistance. This means that the person concerned has probably consumed an excess of carbohydrates over a long period of time. In response, the pancreas has churned out huge amounts of insulin and this makes one hypoglycemic, which means one has a low blood sugar level. The insulin receptors in the pancreas and other parts of the body then become exhausted and fail to respond to the sugar status; the excess sugar builds up in the blood, and diabetes results. When the insulin receptors shut down, insufficient energy is received by the muscles, which then become tired and weak.

If an individual with Type 2 diabetes goes on a good diet and takes a few natural supplements, their diabetes can usually be controlled. One dietary supplement of great benefit here is to take whey powder in the diet, as it is a rich source of glycoprotein.

Type 1 diabetes affects young people, in most cases, and is an autoimmune disease. Here, the individual is more likely to be thin than fat. The cause is unknown, although there is an inherited predisposition in some cases. One theory is that antibodies form after a viral infection in childhood and destroy the pancreatic cells that produce insulin. After a certain number of these cells are destroyed, the pancreas can no longer perform its function of sugar metabolism and sugar builds up in the blood. But, although there is plenty of sugar circulating, the body cannot use it, and the person becomes tired and thin.

Diabetes Case Study: Jenny first visited me at the beginning of 1987, when she was 26. She had been diagnosed with Type 1 diabetes two years before and was depressed about the condition. She also suffered from a depigmentation condition of the skin called vitiligo.

For her first treatment, I gave her zinc, due to its metabolic effect in relation to the pancreas; colloidal sodium sulfate, a cell salt with an affinity with the healthy pancreas; liver and lymphatic toning drops; a homeopathic complex for toning the pancreas; vitamin C for detoxification, and vitamin B complex for energy. Her diabetes stabilized, and she had fewer hypoglycemic attacks following her insulin injections; these are dangerous for diabetics if not corrected with sugar in some form. In recent times, Jenny has been consistently well and the diabetes under control throughout each day.

At times, I have done esoteric healing for diabetes and focused on the digestive triangles and lymphatic drainage for the skin and the nervous system. Sometimes, when doing the energy scan on Jenny, I found the energy in her pancreas disturbed, but other times, it had a normal energy flow.

A year later, Jenny married and her treatment continued mostly unchanged for three years. She got pregnant, after which I added colloidal calcium for the baby's bones and vitamin E to keep the placental circulation in order. A healthy baby was delivered by caesarian section. I prescribed colloidal magnesium and potassium phosphate for the extra energy needed to cope with raising a baby. From a naturopathic perspective, these two tissue salts are the main salts used for the health of the nervous system. It has been found, over the years, that the tissue salt potassium phosphate is helpful in cases of diabetes; this is probably because of the relationship between the autonomic nervous system and all the digestive organs, including the pancreas.

I mentioned earlier that the digestive system can be deficient in energy, causing weak digestion. In the case of juvenile or Type 1 diabetes, we have a special case, in which the antibodies formed, for some reason, attack the tissue in the pancreas that produces insulin. By enhancing the nervous system with potassium phosphate, the remaining healthy cells in the pancreas are strengthened. Later, I switched Jenny to chromium instead of the zinc, as chromium is involved with sugar metabolism; it is also useful for people who put a strain on their pancreas from excessive sugar intake.

Jenny had two more babies at approximately two-year intervals. The medical profession usually advises against a third pregnancy for diabetics, but her third baby was healthy, except for a skin pigmentation condition, which required surgery. Jenny has remained well and continues in a stable condition to this day. She visits every three or four months for a checkup. I am sure that natural therapies over two decades have preserved her health, especially during the pregnancies.

This case shows that, even in chronic conditions like diabetes, there can be a useful synthesis of inner and outer treatment to preserve health. Jenny will always need her insulin injections because the part of the pancreas producing the insulin has been destroyed, but without the natural treatment she would have probably been much worse. This case outcome was chiefly helped by the physical remedies, but I cannot discount the possible energy links to the solar plexus chakra at the time of onset and before the main physical damage to the pancreas took place. Most of the diabetics I have treated in my clinic have come some time after diagnosis and the onset of insulin therapy. I would love to have the chance to use the esoteric treatment at the beginning of the disease, when it would be most useful and more effective to correct any problems in the immune system via the solar plexus and thymus gland—at the energy level first.

The Nervous System and Diarrhea

Diarrhea is one of those ailments closely related to the nervous system and psyche. The sympathetic part of the autonomic nervous system is overstimulated and this prepares us for the fight-or-flight reaction. Therefore, emotions such as fear, panic, and anxiety often cause increased motility and spasm of the intestines, resulting in diarrhea. There is often an accompanying magnesium deficiency. Sometimes I have a client whose severe digestive problems appear to have been largely based on psychological and psychic problems from the past. A dramatic disturbance to the solar plexus and sacral chakras appeared to be the cause for the severe intestinal problem of the next case.

Diarrhea Case Study: Millie, 40, is a trained nurse whose father sexually abused her as a child and teenager. Her symptoms included stress, severe nausea, and diarrhea with pain. At the time of her first visit, she had up to sixteen bowel actions per day. All medical tests for digestive function had proved negative. I found disturbances of the solar plexus chakra, liver, and small and large intestines. Her iris indicated toxic waste in the intestinal area, fanning out into the connective tissues. Many people have a similar level of toxicity without their intestines responding as dramatically as Millie's did.

I prescribed Millie magnesium orotate to slow down the peristaltic movements, and homeopathic drops for the liver and lymphatic system. I gave her Bach flower essences for her emotional state: Star of Bethlehem for shock, Cherry Plum for desperation, Mimulus for fear, Hornbeam for strength, Walnut to break her links with the past, Heather for an overconcern with self, and Gorse for hopelessness. Millie's naturopathic treatment varied monthly, depending on her health changes. I added a digestive mixture after the bowel actions had settled; as herbs can be too strong when the digestion is severely disturbed, I initially used homeopathic remedies. After ten days of treatment, her bowel actions reduced from sixteen per day to seven, and after a few months of treatment were down to two or three daily.

The chakras that were mainly affected in Millie's condition were the solar plexus and sacral. My energy scan revealed persistent thought-forms affecting the sacral center, probably because of the sexual abuse. I was not sure whether the psychiatric counseling she received was doing any good or just encouraging morbid reflections on the problem. She had one bad psychological relapse that led to an admission for psychiatric treatment, as she felt suicidal. Following that episode, she has continually improved; her energy has remained good, and she is now back to work as a nurse. Intermittently she needs to take pharmaceutical medication.

As I have outlined earlier, esoteric healing lifts the eyes of the personality off the problem area and into the soul. This is a different approach from delving into and bringing to the surface all the traumas of the past, as was the approach of her psychiatrist. So there is the more orthodox approach of delving into the past and alternatively, an approach where we bypass the past and focus on the healing energies of the soul, to wipe out the negative associations of the past that are conditioning one's health.

If we spell out more clearly the reaction of Millie to sexual abuse by her father, we could suggest that despite suppression of this abuse for decades, her personality had walled off the experience; even so, it was waiting to come up for resolution. So, after certain triggers, these incest experiences surfaced and needed to be resolved. During this period, the chakras affected were the sacral (which relates to the sexual organs and lower part of the large bowel) and the solar plexus (which expresses our emotions including fear). It is a common experience that fear causes increased bowel movements and, in this case, there were sixteen per day. The accompanying nausea probably related to the fact that, as a child, she had to cope with her father's penis being forced down her throat on a regular basis.

The esoteric healing during this reliving process was given to stabilize the intense activity of the sacral and solar plexus while Millie grappled with these memories. It was also intended to help Millie lift her emotions and thoughts (the "eyes of the personality") off the past and to align herself with the healing energies flowing from her soul.

In Millie's case, the two approaches, orthodox and esoteric, seem to have been very positive, as she had no relapse of the nausea, diarrhea, or headaches. I used the digestive triangles, shock triangle, vagus triangle, and aspirant's triangle. As with all esoteric healing treatments, I make minor variations each time, depending on what is happening in the client's life. With all clients, I encourage them to attend my meditation classes, and some choose to do the healing courses. If this is not possible, I give them one of my meditation tapes.

Chronic Bowel Disorders

In addition to the causes of poor digestion already described, there are also inherited predispositions and autoimmune disorders of the digestive system such as ulcerative colitis. Ulcerative colitis features severe inflammation of the large colon and may, in part, result from the action of destructive antibodies. Crohn's disease is another autoimmune condition that usually affects the small intestines and causes thickening of the mucous membrane, resulting in pain, spasm, and sometimes blockage. It can be associated also with arthritis, as in the following case. This case is of interest because I treated Louise before and through her second pregnancy. The baby was delivered safely and in a healthy condition, despite Louise needing large amounts of cortisone throughout much of her pregnancy.

Crohn's Disease Case Study: Louise, 33, first visited me in the winter of 1996; she had suffered Crohn's Disease for many years and was on 30 mg of cortisone per day. As well as her bowel problems, she had joint pains in her knees and ankles, and she was tired, but she was not suffering diarrhea while on this large amount of cortisone. Her iris indicated heavy lymphatic congestion and a moderate degree of acidity; the autonomic nervous system was imbalanced; and the etheric scan revealed disturbed energy in the lymphatic system and small intestine.

Her first prescription included an herbal tablet for lymphatic cleansing with burdock, red clover, poke root, and echinacea; homeopathic drops for lymphatic and liver cleansing; a tablet with anti-inflammatory herbs for the joints; zinc to deal with the adhesions in the small bowel; and colloidal sodium phosphate to reduce the acidity throughout her tissues.

On her return visit after one month, Louise reported more vitality, although her right eye had become blurry; the right knee became swollen after her cortisone had been reduced to 20 mg per day. When I did an energy scan, I discovered that the adrenal glands indicated an energy disturbance; this was understandable, as the cortisone was now reduced and they needed to work harder. I added support for the adrenal glands in the form of vitamin B_5, homeopathic drops, and vitamin C.

After this second visit, Louise felt much better but, unfortunately, she did not continue treatment. She returned six months later, having suffered an abdominal abscess and a temporary ileostomy. An ileostomy means an opening into the small intestine, in this case, to rest the large intestine, so that the daily stools are temporarily excreted through the abdominal wall, allowing the large intestine to recover from its intense inflammation. The ileostomy had been undone before her next visit to me, the abdominal opening had been closed, and the pieces of intestine joined together again. An energy scan showed significant disturbance in her intestines. She had had no menstruation for several months, which indicated the general upset to her whole system. She felt the abscess was recurring, as she started to suffer symptoms similar to before it was treated.

When I scanned her etheric field, I found considerable disturbance in the abdominal area, and the solar plexus was larger than the other chakras, indicating a possible blockage that was affecting the organs in the abdominal area. I was concerned that the abscess might be returning. After balancing all the chakras so that the solar plexus was relieved of congestion, I did the vitality triangles and then the lymphatic drainage technique for her abdominal area. This was to move the toxins along the lymphatic channels and through the lymphatic glands more adequately and to relieve the stasis of toxins that was building towards another abscess.

After the healing, I gave Louise 2 g of echinacea per day and 4 g of vitamin C to boost her immune system; I repeated the zinc to assist the wound healing; and iron phosphate, potassium chloride, and calcium sulfate in colloidal form to prevent a new abscess from forming.

On her return visit, Louise reported that her menstruation had resumed the day after the last visit. Her abdominal area was still throbbing a bit, but an ultrasound revealed no further development of an abscess. I continued her treatment and gave her vitamin E to help with the wound healing. A month later, she still had a sharp pain in the area where the abscess had originally manifested. Her periods had become regular and her eyelashes had grown back. Their earlier disappearance was an indication of the autoimmune aspect of her disease. After another month of treatment, the abdominal pain had gone completely but she still had abdominal bloating. She was concerned about her weight, as she had gained 21 pounds in six months.

I adjusted her treatment to include the herb euphrasia ("eye bright") in her drops for the continuing discomfort in her eye; I gave her homeopathic charcoal for the bloating and flatulence; and progesterone extract from wild yam to be used topically for the bloating, as this preparation helps balance the hormones which, when imbalanced, cause fluid retention and swelling of the abdomen. Her herbal rheumatic tablet was continued. The next month, she started having problems again with diarrhea, so I added magnesium orotate (400 mg twice daily) to her prescription. I also gave her silica in colloidal form to break up her bowel adhesions that were giving some discomfort with a pulling sensation. I continued the esoteric healing at each office visit.

After nine months of treatment, and times when her health seemed to be going backwards into renewed abdominal discomfort, Louise started to have alternating months where she was fairly good, in terms of both bowel and joints. Sometimes the bowel relapsed with inflammation and pain, and I would find energy disturbances in the area of discomfort. At other times, her energy seemed balanced. She sometimes came for extra healing between her normal monthly visits, and she always felt much better after the healing. Even so, she still needed to be on large doses of cortisone sometimes, as well as having this full naturopathic treatment regimen.

The list of Louise's naturopathic medicines stayed fairly constant for a while, and included an herbal mixture for the intestines that featured meadowsweet, red clover, chelidonium, chamomile, marshmallow root, and a dash of goldenseal; magnesium orotate for bowel spasm; silica in colloidal form for possible abdominal adhesions; liver and lymph cleansing drops; and colloidal potassium phosphate for energy. Throughout her treatment, she continued taking a vitamin B complex that she had started before my treatment.

Towards the end of 1997, Louise decided that she was well enough to get pregnant. I thought this move was a bit premature, but did not interfere and she became pregnant at the beginning of 1998. We started a concerted effort to keep her well during her pregnancy. At three months of pregnancy, she was on 17.5 mg of cortisone, which increased to 60 mg daily at one stage; with this in mind, one of my main aims was to provide the growing baby with enough vitamins and minerals for its health, despite the drug therapy.

A further complication occurred (apart from increasing joint problems): psoriasis. This troublesome skin disease is characterized by large oval and scaling red patches: Louise had these all over her legs. This disease was a further indication of the autoimmune dimension to her problems. Her treatment had to be changed to accommodate this skin problem, and her mixture was altered to include herbs that work on the immune system, such as echinacea, catmint, and cat's claw. I also kept her on some of the digestive herbs.

I discovered, when doing the esoteric healing, that her thyroid gland was now underactive, so I added kelp tablets and homeopathic kelp to her regimen. The magnesium orotate was continued, and so was the extract of yam cream to keep up her progesterone levels. Around this time, I started to use "Noni Juice" from Tahiti (derived from a tree) with clients with serious problems that had not fully responded to naturopathic treatment. This natural plant product seemed to have a very good effect on Louise, and her joints and skin improved at last, after which the herbal mixture was discontinued.

Towards the end of her pregnancy, she developed a large cyst on the thyroid gland. This may have been caused by the huge doses of cortisone she took throughout her pregnancy. Fortunately, the cortisone was being tapered off at this stage, although she was still very puffy in the face and body from its use.

A healthy baby was delivered in late August, and I was amazed to find that the iris of this baby showed a good constitution, despite Louise's problems throughout the pregnancy and her constant medication with cortisone. Louise continued treatment for some time after the birth of the baby and was off her cortisone, with no ill effects. Louise remained well without either medical or naturopathic aid. The baby had a very healthy development. She has continued in excellent health and attributes this to taking regular supplements of glyconutrients plus a nutrient formula including antioxidants. Her Crohn's disease has remained in remission; she has lost weight, and is now pregnant again with no problems; her two-year-old daughter is also in excellent health.

Louise's is a good case to indicate that perseverance pays off. This case is somewhat the reverse of the previous one, inasmuch as I could not detect any negative influence from her psyche influencing her condition. The problem seemed to be directly in the physical/etheric field and had worked *back into* the associated chakra—the solar plexus. The interaction of the psyche and body does not cause every health problem.

In a longstanding problem of a physical nature, there will be disturbance working back into the associated chakras at the etheric level, in contrast to a case where negative thoughts and feelings condition the etheric chakras. Louise became pregnant very easily when the abdominal symptoms were partly resolved, and I think this is probably another indication that the problem was local, meaning that there were no specific underlying psychological causes.

Colon Cancer

From a naturopathic viewpoint, colon cancer is an example of the final stage of digestive problems. This cancer often spreads to the liver, and is a major cause of death in Western countries, accounting for 20% of all cancer deaths. Poor diet is a major cause, and medical authorities now urge us to have plenty of fiber in our diet, as in wholemeal breads, salads, vegetables, and fruits. Research indicates that carrots, green vegetables such as broccoli, and beets provide particular factors that are preventive against cancer.

I see colon cancer as having multiple causes, but, clearly, poor nutrition ranks high in the concern of natural therapists. There are two aspects to the nutrition question:

First, there is the accumulation of toxic substances from refined foods such as white flour and sugar products; the thousands of chemicals added to foods as flavorings, colorings, emulsifiers, and preservatives; rancid oils and fats in fast foods, where the same oil has been used for days; and carcinogenic products like aspartame that are allowed as artificial sweeteners in some countries.

Second is an antioxidant deficiency. Antioxidants preserve cell membranes by acting as scavengers for the free radicals that cause the damage. Examples of foods containing antioxidants are fruits and vegetables that contain large amounts of vitamins C and E. However, since most of our fruits and vegetables come to us after cold storage, it is very difficult to obtain sufficient vitamin C, for instance, without supplementation. The vitamin C content of fruit and vegetables disappears with most types storage. The preservation of vitamin E is just as difficult, for once a cereal or nut is broken or cut, the product must be consumed almost immediately or the vitamin E is destroyed.

Another important cause for colon cancer, recognized by the medical profession, is chronic constipation caused by poor diets. A diet high in dietary fiber and complex carbohydrates is found to reduce the risk of colorectal (colon and rectal) cancer.[39] Vegetarians, who generally have a diet high in fruits, vegetables, and wholegrain cereals have reduced rates of colorectal cancer.[40] I have cited some other causes for constipation earlier in the chapter, and these causes include spasm in the solar plexus and/or sacral center, sluggish thyroid function, and general exhaustion of the digestive system.

In some cases, there is an inherited factor for cancer, but a recent research paper based on a study of thousands of identical twins did not find a very high percentage of bowel cancer in the twins. It was under 5%, so it seems that lifestyle and other factors must be more important.

From an esoteric perspective, we will be studying the state of the solar plexus and sacral chakras, in relation to bowel cancer. These chakras may be blocked through suppression of negative emotions, such as anger in its suppressed form as resentment. I have found that many of my bowel cancer patients do not express their emotions freely and are inclined to hang on to hurts. This prevents a free flow of energy through their chakras. There is usually an inner (subjective) and an outer (objective) factor involved in most chronic disease, but individuals who have not suppressed their negative emotions may, perhaps, have other chronic diseases, but not cancer. This is a generalization because there are forms of cancer that are more or less inevitable, such as that resulting from extreme radiation exposure.

We also meet psychologically balanced individuals who seem to get away with a dreadful diet throughout their life and yet seem to be immune from most cancers, including colorectal malignancies. This may indicate again that we need both an inner and outer factor for cancer to develop. If the energies are flowing freely through the chakras from our subjective life, then outer factors, such as environmental toxins and poor diet, may be better tolerated (see the case of George under lymphatic problems).

In holistic medicine I consider it the challenge of the physician to establish which is most predominant, the inner or outer factors of each case. As we go through the various cases in this book, note that I have mentioned in some cases that the inner or outer factors are most prominent. In many cases, there are strong physical *and* emotional factors.

Colon Cancer Case Study: Robert had a fairly colorful health history that began when he was fourteen years old with an abscessed appendix. During his hospital stay for an appendectomy, he had an epileptic fit and was later diagnosed with the typical brain pattern suggesting the need of lifelong drugs for epilepsy. Perhaps as a prelude to his later bowel cancer, he had an early tendency, when he became emotionally disturbed, to bowel upsets, in the form of diarrhea. He stated that, according to his parents, even as a child he tended to be a loner and often retired to his room in an introverted state rather than mention why he was upset. His diarrhea was sometimes followed by an epileptic fit, despite taking medication for epilepsy.

Reflecting on this history from an esoteric perspective, I concluded that Robert probably had a disturbance in his sacral and solar plexus chakras from an early age, and that this related to his fairly suppressed emotional upsets and the diarrhea tendency. Robert studied interior design after leaving school and, in his twenties, went overseas to work. When he was about thirty, he had malignant nodules on his thyroid and his thyroid was removed by radiation; thus his medication had to then include thyroxine, the thyroid hormone. Now you might ask what the epilepsy or thyroid has to do with bowel cancer. Apart from the connection of a suppressed emotional life with solar plexus and sacral disturbance, the sacral and throat chakras are energetically connected. It is likely Robert's sacral/throat axis was disturbed from an early age, causing problems in relation to both chakras later.

For most of his life before developing the bowel cancer, Robert had a serious drinking problem, and he stopped drinking three years before his cancer was diagnosed, following dire warnings from his doctor. The drinking problem was another indication of solar plexus and sacral center imbalances. At the time of giving up drinking, he separated from his partner of ten years and had to sell his luxury flat and move to a more modest apartment due to a job change. There were, therefore, a lot of problems to further upset his chakras, especially the solar plexus, which relates to our emotional life. As he used to be a senior consultant in interior design, it was a blow to his self-esteem to be downgraded.

During the three years before being diagnosed with cancer, he lost a large amount of weight, but all tests, including a colonoscopy, were negative. The tumor was hard to find, because it was located near the caecum—blind pouch near the appendix. Just before I started treating Robert, he had emergency surgery for a hemorrhaging colon cancer; he was 58. The surgery was successful; it was followed by chemotherapy, and then he was treated by me.

From the physical point of view, his liver had been under stress, having to deal with his epilepsy and thyroid drugs plus the alcohol intake over several decades. This meant the liver would be less able to cope with carcinogens taken into his body. I gave Robert the following prescription as soon as he came out of hospital: vitamin C (2 g per day); an herbal tablet containing cat's claw, astragalus, goldenseal, and olive leaf for detoxification and immune support; vitamin E (300 IU) and a zinc tablet for wound healing; liver and lymphatic toning homeopathic drops; grapeseed extract (60 mg) as a further antioxidant to support the vitamin C; and potassium phosphate and magnesium phosphate in colloidal form for balancing the nervous system.

Robert also received esoteric healing to balance his chakras, cleanse the lymphatic system, and boost the immune system (see description of the immune triangle), and the digestive system was regulated with the digestive triangles. Initially, following surgery, I found the chakras to be weak and lacking in energy, but they returned to normal strength surprisingly quickly. I also spent time teaching Robert to meditate (see appendix 2) and gave him a tape, by which he could practice daily at home. He found meditation difficult once he went back to work. He was fortunate that a colon resection was able to be performed, that a colostomy was not needed, and that his scar healed very well. His oncologist arranged for chemotherapy to start after a few weeks. Robert stayed with a relative who helped look after his postoperative needs, and, after a few weeks, he was back at his new but, in his view, dreary drafting job.

He managed to keep working throughout the weeks of his chemotherapy, and looked after himself and his cats at home. Gradually, he restored himself to health. His nausea during the chemotherapy was minimal, and he did not lose his hair. It is remarkable how natural therapies can help the body cope during chemotherapy.

From time to time, I changed his natural remedies. After about a year of the herbal therapy, I replaced it with the bovine tracheal cartilage, which not only prevents cancer cell spread but also helps reduce the inflammation of joints. This was indicated because Robert was having a lot of trouble with lower back pain at the time. He continued with all the other treatments.

The oncologist reported to Robert that he had needed the chemotherapy because his cancer had invaded some of the abdominal lymphatic glands. After the chemotherapy finished, Robert had the usual six-month checkups, and his oncologist was very pleased with his progress. His liver function tests have returned to normal, and he has remained off alcohol now for six years. It is now four years since his surgery; he appears to be in excellent health, and is thinking of retiring to a country town.

This is a good case to illustrate the part played by both subjective and outer factors in the life over several decades. The inner factors of early emotional disturbance were fairly significant for Robert and conditioned his sacral and solar plexus chakras, which added to some disturbance already in the throat chakra from an early age. The outer factors included the effects on the liver of heavy alcohol consumption and the need for the liver to detoxify his other drugs. In terms of the chakras, Robert is much more stabilized and is philosophical about his life situation and future possibilities, and the state of his chakras reflect his newfound stability.

Most people have a tremendous fear about cancer, and this emotion in itself can cause us to be predisposed to cancer because energy follows thought. We should look at the gastrointestinal tract as remaining or becoming healthy in proportion to the health of both our physical and psychic assimilation and elimination. We can consider assimilation as not only of our physical food and drink but of our emotions, thoughts, and psychic impacts from our daily encounters. If we have a healthy way of dealing with this more subtle "food" and can eliminate psychological waste, our physical digestion will tend to be healthy and resistant to disease.

We should look at the gastrointestinal tract as remaining or becoming healthy in proportion to the health of both our physical and psychic assimilation and elimination. We can consider assimilation as not only of our physical food and drink but of our emotions, thoughts, and psychic impacts from our daily encounters.

Language has an interesting way of expressing our subtle states. Someone will say, "I can't *stomach* that," meaning they cannot assimilate a particular situation. We need to address all the factors for health in these areas and to understand that no one factor will cause digestive problems. We need to consume healthy food and water; entertain healthy emotions and thoughts (an endeavor assisted greatly by meditation); and use the many self-help systems now available.

By way of review, let's recall that we started our practical journey through some of the health conditions related to the solar plexus because that is the first chakra to balance in the healing process. These solar plexus conditions are the digestive disorders commonly encountered in my practice, and I have endeavored to show here how a synthesis of therapies, including physical medicine and esoteric treatment, can best treat the whole person. I have also indicated how there may be a variable emphasis on either the inner or outer factors in a given case.

The effects of psychic and nervous stress on our solar plexus chakra have been discussed, as well as the subsequent effect on our digestion, depending on whether the solar plexus partly shuts down or becomes too open. We need to lift the "eyes of the personality" (emotions and thoughts) off the problem area and allow the healing energies of the soul to flow in.

We will now look at the practical work and triangles associated with these case histories for digestive problems, so that you are equipped to use these exercises on yourself and others. Remember that the healing will be successful in proportion to your inner alignment with the soul. Daily meditation will be a great help to maintain alignment to your inner essence; a suitable format for this is described in appendix 2. Also, by doing some kind of alignment or centering on a daily basis, the alignment process with a client is enhanced.

If you are working on yourself, imagine during the healing that your etheric body is sitting in front of you, and carry out the same procedure as if there was a physical body of another person on the chair. The same process can be used when healing another person at a distance. Alternatively, when healing yourself, you, as the healer, can imagine that your energy body is sitting sideways on your lap for the chakra balancing; then turn this energy body around to face you when doing the triangles.

Healing Practice for the Solar Plexus and the Digestive System

1. Align with the soul described in part 1: place your hands on the client's shoulders and imagine linking up with your own soul, the client's soul, and the source of all healing, and ask that healing take place according to the plan of the soul.

2. Visualize the healer's flow of energy by imagining the following alignment: soul, heart, head, and hands.

3. When you sense that the energies are flowing, move to the left-hand side of the client and kneel or sit so that you can comfortably have your hands on either side of their body. From this point on, you do not physically need to touch the client.

4. Balance all the chakras up the spine (as described earlier) by placing your right hand behind the spine of the client and your left hand in front. Sense the impact of the energies on your hands, and move them gently in and out, in an accordion fashion, until the flow of energies seems balanced between your two hands. Balance the chakras in the order of solar plexus, base, sacral, heart, and throat. During this process, there is no need to have the hands close to the body. It is best to have them as far away as possible, because it seems to be easier to assess the energies in this way and is less disturbing to the client.

5. Move in front of the client and, from a distance of a few feet, imagine connecting your brow chakra with the solar plexus of the client and connect your palm chakras with the liver and liver minor center (see figure 10). Imagine connecting the three points of solar plexus, liver organ, and liver minor center with light, then visualize the whole triangle to be filled with light. Wait a few moments until the energy is stabilized.

6. Make a second triangle by keeping your brow center focused on the solar plexus and use your hand chakras to connect with the stomach and stomach minor chakra.

7. Visualize three points of solar plexus, stomach organ, and stomach minor chakra to be connected by a triangle of light. Fill the triangle with light (see figure 11). You do not need to see the lines of light in a physical sense, as it is sufficient to imagine the quality of light linking the three points.

8. The third triangle connects the three digestive organs of pancreas, liver, and stomach. So move your brow center to focus on the pancreas while one palm center connects with the liver of the client and the other palm center with the client's stomach (see figure 12).

The Digestive Triangles. The digestive triangles are useful to visualize for all digestive disorders. The energy flows from the solar plexus chakra through all the digestive organs more serenely. The solar plexus chakra is always balanced first.

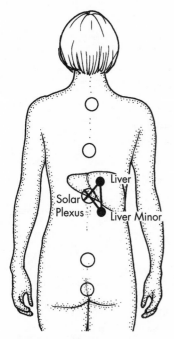

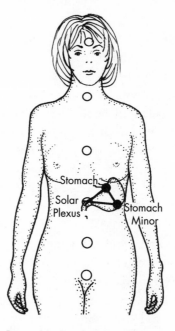

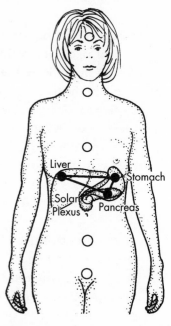

FIGURE 10: THE LIVER TRIANGLE. The liver triangle is used for all liver and gallbladder disturbances or disease. The healer vitalizes the triangle by connecting, in imagination, their brow chakra and palm chakra with these three points.

FIGURE 11: THE STOMACH TRIANGLE. The stomach triangle is used for all stomach and digestive ailments. The healer vitalizes this triangle by connecting, in imagination, their brow chakra with solar plexus, one hand chakra with the stomach organ and the other hand chakra with the stomach minor chakra.

FIGURE 12: THE STOMACH, LIVER, AND PANCREAS TRIANGLE. As with the other digestive triangles, the healer vitalizes this triangle by connecting three points within their own energy field—brow chakra and both hand chakras—with the liver, stomach, and pancreas.

9. Close the aura of the client by using your hands or imagination to make the shape of an oval around the client, from the feet upwards, with a gentle sweeping motion. Imagine gently withdrawing the healing energy back through your hands to your soul, so as to break the connection with the client now that the healing is completed.

10. Visualize closing up your own aura in whatever way seems best. To do this, you can imagine using the same movement on yourself as has been used for the client.

   The reason that we close the aura is because the healing process opens the client to becoming more sensitive to any physical or psychic impact. If, after the healing, the person goes into a noisy and busy environment, the good effect of the healing could not only be lost, but they may feel nervy and disturbed. The same applies to you as the healer. It is preferable, after any healing, for the client to be able to remain in a quiet environment for as long as possible, so that the healing work can be grounded into their energy field. The healer should preferably wash their own hands after the healing.

You will note that, during the healing process, a number of triangles have also been made by the healer. These assist the flow of energies. For example, there is the initial triangle within the healer during the alignment process between the soul, heart, and head with an extension to the hands. While visualizing each triangle on the client, the healer makes a triangle between her brow center and hand chakras.

8 The Base Chakra and Musculo-Skeletal Problems

The next chakra to be balanced in our healing protocol is the base or root chakra. It is appropriately placed after digestive conditions, because our metabolic processes have a big influence on our muscles and skeletal system, and especially on the spine, which, together with the adrenal glands and kidneys, is related to this chakra.

The base chakra is the second chakra we balance in the healing protocol. You may remember that it relates to the spine, kidneys, and bladder, and, indirectly, to the muscles. It is obviously related in some ways to the Earth and to our capacity for "grounding." In other words, if this chakra is weak, the energy in our whole body suffers and it is difficult to stand straight and keep the spine erect. If you observe people in a shopping center, you will notice how few people stand straight—they are bent in all directions, especially the elderly. If you measured the size of their chakras and energy flow through their chakras, you would find the base center is often energetically weak.

Spinal problems are almost endemic. I recently attended a healing conference, at which the lecturer asked all those with back trouble in the audience to stand up; two-thirds of the audience rose. So in this chapter, we will explore the conditions associated with an unbalanced base chakra, the associated tissues of skeleton, muscles, kidneys, and their esoteric and naturopathic implications.

The base chakra is associated with the will to live and be. You may remember that the endocrine glands associated with the base chakra are the adrenals, which sit like little caps on top of the kidneys. In keeping with the base chakra characteristics, their secretions of adrenalin and cortisone are also associated with life-threatening ill-nesses such as severe allergic reactions and also for chronic ailments like rheumatoid arthritis and other serious skeletal problems.

As with most health disorders discussed in this book, we cannot isolate the cases mentioned in this chapter as being related to the base chakra alone. For instance, rheumatoid arthritis will often have thymus gland disturbances relating to the heart chakra, and an imbal-ance of the solar plexus associated with poor diet may also predispose some individuals to arthritis of various types.

When dealing with skeletal problems, I frequently combine Bowen Therapy with esoteric healing and find that this synthesis, together with particular supplements, is very complementary. The esoteric healing seems to help the Bowen Therapy to be immediately effective, instead of it taking perhaps hours or days to resolve musculo-skeletal problems.

From a physical and naturopathic view, our skeletons are under constant renewal from wear and tear throughout our lives, and they suffer severely if our nutrition is not adequate. Most people think of taking calcium as the main requirement for maintaining bone health, but other substances may be more important. Magnesium is essential for tensile strength and, as mentioned earlier, it is seriously lacking in the modern diet. Zinc is another important mineral nutrient for the bones. Vitamin C is needed for all connective tissue, including bones; vitamins A and D are also needed, the latter for calcium absorption. We also need vitamin E for mobility of ligaments and tendons. Boron is a trace element needed to prevent arthritis, but it has been largely ignored in this context until recently.

The types of musculo-skeletal conditions that can be helped by natural therapies and esoteric healing include osteoporosis, all kinds of arthritis, disc degeneration, the healing of fractures, and muscular conditions such as fibromyalgia.

Causes of Skeletal Problems

A lot of spinal and joint problems relate to tensions in the sur-rounding muscles, ligaments, and tendons. I find that many tensions in the muscles and ligaments have subtle causes. Mention has been made as to the interrelation between the chakras. I find that the muscles and ligaments around the sacral center or sacroiliac joint on the physical body are often very tense; this tension can relate to sacral center issues such as money or sex. The fears and worries associated with the solar plexus center as the gateway to the emotions will also cause tensions in the musculature. Moving further up the spine, "cerebral" people who think excessively often have great tension in the large muscle across the top of the body called the trapezius, as well as problems with the cervical vertebrae in the neck.

From a physical perspective, magnesium is needed to prevent tension in the connective tissue.[41] As this is the most commonly deficient mineral (as found in my practice), I am constantly supplementing clients with muscular skeletal problems with magnesium orotate, magnesium phosphate, or magnesium chelate. I find that the fascial (muscle covering) therapy or Bowen technique is a valuable and noninvasive way of balancing energies across the musculature, and that this returns the skeleton to normal positioning. Most of the points on the body used in Bowen Therapy relate to acupuncture points, so it seems we may be working with the Chinese meridian system in this approach.

When thinking about muscular and skeletal problems, we have two main issues—spasms caused by mineral deficiencies and psychic stress, plus immobility caused by adhesions and degeneration. From the inner side, immobility is often due to some rigid traits in the personality, and this will be mirrored in the ligaments and joints. If we keep a flexible mind, it can be mirrored in our body. Considering the physical aspect, any joint can become immobilized if the smooth hyaline cartilage covering the joint breaks down and adhesions start to form from the underlying spongier bone. This process can happen if the connective tissues become too acidic from poor diet, metabolism, or stress; in many cases, these are triggering factors for inherited tendencies to manifest. Whether the process is called osteoarthritis or some other name, the same subtle and physical treatment often helps.

However, muscular and skeletal conditions generally take a long time to resolve, due to the density of the ligaments, tendons, and joints as compared with other body tissues. In addition, pain often only develops after there has been considerable degeneration. From an esoteric perspective, blocks in the psyche are often related to a stiffening or thickening of one kind or another in the skeleton, ligaments, and joints of the body. Therefore, naturopathic treatment, psychological work, and esoteric healing are appropriate measures that may be needed over a long period of time.

Osteoarthritis

All forms of arthritis have a combination of causes from a holistic perspective. There is usually an inherited tendency, triggered by stress and/or poor diet. Osteoarthritis often affects the large joints in a singular fashion—shoulder, hip, knee, wrist. One of the most common expressions of this malady in postmenopausal women are Heberdeen nodes, swellings on the terminal phalanges (joints) of the fingers. They can be so large that many activities using the hands become very painful. Any form of arthritis can take a long time to respond, just as it takes many years for the conditions to develop.

The general esoteric aspect of immobilized joints has been mentioned, but the possible inner cause for the formation of Heberdeen nodes is interesting. I find women with these problems often confirm my instinct that their creative energies are blocked; ideally, these energies should be flowing from the throat center and down the arms, to be expressed in some creative way in the world.

The diet is very important in the physical treatment of this condition, as an acidic diet with few fresh vegetables and salads can cause the calcium in the body to get out of balance and form deposits around the joints. I often suggest that clients take two glasses of raw juices daily, consisting of equal parts of carrot, apple, and celery, and half this amount of beet. The iris often reveals that the sufferer of arthritis has experienced poor elimination through the bowel for many years.

We can bring in the esoteric side here, and reflect on how the solar plexus chakra is also involved with skeletal problems. For if our desires for junk food, as conditioned by the solar plexus, predominate, then the skeleton will suffer eventually from mineral imbalance. For instance, if the tissues become acidic as a result of poor diet, calcium will be deposited in the wrong places, causing adhesions and calcification. The possible inherited factors for arthritis can be addressed with high potency homeopathic remedies.

Hip degeneration is probably the most common among major joint problems that I encounter but, unfortunately, most clients in this category only come to my clinic at the stage when they need a hip replacement. If they took treatment at the first sign of degeneration, then a lot could be done to halt, and even reverse, such degeneration. Spinal disc degeneration is also very common and, again, it can be halted, and even reversed, if a client is willing to persevere with at least two years of treatment. There are a number of supplements that can keep joints healthy and reverse damage, if not too extensive.

For example, glucosamine and chondroitin sulfate can gradually lubricate and restore joint processes, if used over six months or more. Anti-inflammatory herbs and the antioxidant vitamins C and E have profound effects on connective tissue and joint mobility, respectively. Other elements, such as manganese, are necessary for healthy joints and discs. Homeopathic silica can gradually break up adhesions, but it takes a long time. Magnesium may be needed for spasm of ligaments and tendons. The client's nutrition must be examined, to ascertain whether the diet is sufficiently alkaline to keep calcium in balance.

The esoteric healing for skeletal problems will include the opening triangles associated with the throat chakra, shoulders, and arms; the grounding triangles associated with the sacral center and legs, and the adrenal triangle associated with the base center and adrenal glands. There are also techniques for moving energy up the spine to correct spinal misalignments for those who do the esoteric healing training (see exercise at the end of this chapter).

A Case of Frozen Shoulder: Frozen shoulder is probably one of the most common osteoarthritic problems in joints. This next case is an outstanding example of what can be achieved with holistic therapy. Michelle, 50, visited me for a number of problems, notably obesity that had rapidly increased since menopause, but which started when she began using the contraceptive pill years earlier. She was suffering hot flushes and low libido, and had suffered a frozen shoulder for years, with severe accompanying pain day and night. She had suffered menopause symptoms for fifteen years, since the age of thirty-five, which indicated, from my clinical perspective, that the contraceptive pill had a very unbalancing effect on her hormonal status.

One esoteric cause for her continuing problems related to the emotional shock of a physical attack from one of her male students at the college where she taught. This took place not long before her shoulder condition worsened. We can see here a connection between a disturbance to the base chakra with its relation to the survival instinct and her attack, after which the shoulder worsened. A weakened base center could easily be reflected in parts of the skeleton that are already disturbed in some way.

Her iris revealed a moderate level of toxins, fanning out from the digestive tract into the connective tissues. A scan of her energy field revealed right ovary and thyroid disturbances, endocrine imbalances, which would fit in with both the weight gain and postmenopausal symptoms. It was interesting that blood tests had not revealed a thyroid problem. I often find that an energy scan discerns disturbances before they register on a blood test. Michelle's first prescription included anti-inflammatory herbs, homeopathic drops for liver, lymph glands, and thyroid, the nerve toning tissue salts potassium and magnesium phosphate, and the progesterone-promoting cream from wild yam. I also did the Bowen Therapy for her back and shoulders, and combined it with esoteric healing.

In addition to the base center balancing, the esoteric healing focused on the chakras governing the thyroid (throat) and ovaries (sacral), because the associated organs were found disturbed with the energy scan. Apart from the chakra balance, the other need was to correct the energy in the minor chakra at her right shoulder, so I used the opening triangles, because they involve the shoulders and arms—throat chakra and shoulder minor centers, throat and elbow minors, throat and hand minors (see appendix 1). The Bowen technique, I have found, seems to work much more quickly when followed by the subtle healing techniques.

Michelle called about three days later, to say that she could not believe the improvement in her shoulder. The pain had gone completely and she had much more movement. As it was certainly too early for the supplements to be working, this improvement must be attributed to the Bowen Therapy and healing session; in the long term, though, the remedies would be important to correct the other problems mentioned and to consolidate her shoulder improvement. On her return visit after a month, Michelle was continuing to do well although the hot flushes had not gone. I advised that she double the dosage of wild yam cream and repeat the overall treatment prescription. An energy scan revealed that the corrections to the disturbances were being maintained.

A month later, the flushes were reduced and her shoulder was continuing to get better. Weight was slowly dropping off. After fifteen years of hormone imbalance, any weight loss is bound to take a long time. An energy scan revealed that the ovaries and thyroid continued to stay in balance. The Bowen and esoteric healing therapies were repeated.

I enjoyed working with Michelle. Although she came to the clinic with a lot of problems, she had a positive attitude, and this is very important, especially for getting an optimal effect from esoteric healing. Her shoulder problem, weight, energy, and libido issues all improved during the first six months of treatment, and she got a new job, which improved her career prospects.

From the esoteric perspective, it was significant that the problem areas were linked. The throat center, with its endocrine gland, the thyroid, governs metabolism and therefore weight gain, and also governs the shoulders. So we see how, in Michelle, both the weight gain and shoulder were problems linked through her throat chakra. The menopause symptoms related to the disturbed ovarian energy, and the ovaries, as we know, are ruled by the sacral center. The libido is also related to the sacral and base centers, and this improved as the energies became more balanced. Michelle is continuing treatment at the rate of once every two or three months, and her improvement has been maintained for six months now.

A Case of Osteoarthritis: The next case involves an older woman who also had multiple problems. Both she and her daughter have base chakra problems that manifest in the associated glands, the adrenals. The crux of her joint problem was probably the weakness of the base center, as it is related to the cortisone level of the body as secreted by the adrenals.

There was also sluggish energy in the thyroid, and this can so often cause stasis in the joints. In every case of immobile joints, I would say that there is frozen energy and very often this is partly related to the thyroid chakra with its relation to creativity. The throat chakra relates

> *So we see how, in Michelle, both the weight gain and shoulder were problems linked through her throat chakra. The menopause symptoms related to the disturbed ovarian energy, and the ovaries, as we know, are ruled by the sacral center.*

to the concrete mind, planning, and designing. If the energy does not flow through it easily, there will be possible blockages of energy affecting the metabolism and joints, as the next case with Grace shows. Grace's library work was typical of regimental activity that lacks creativity, expressions of which are needed for a healthy throat chakra.

Grace, 68, just retired as a librarian, has suffered osteoarthritis for many years, and has been consulting me for four years. Her problem came on quite suddenly, eighteen months prior to having treatment at my clinic. Her shoulders, neck, upper arms, and hips were affected. She had headaches from the neck problems, and previous medical treatment made her bowels sluggish. Her mother had mild arthritic problems.

Her iris showed a heavy level of toxic waste in the body, including lymphatic congestion. There were also nerve rings, indicating the need for the nerve tissue salts. When I scanned the energy field, I found disturbed energy in the thymus gland, kidneys, adrenal glands, and lymphatic glands. A disturbance in the thymus usually indicates an autoimmune problem.

Previous medical treatment for Grace had included a low dose of cortisone, anti-inflammatory drugs, diuretics, and thyroxine (thyroid hormone) over a six-year period for an underactive thyroid. The underactive thyroid is typical in cases of lack of creativity, due to a lack of energy flowing through the throat center. Her naturopathic treatment included anti-inflammatory herbs such as guaiacum and burdock; homeopathic liver and lymph drops for cleansing and toning those tissues; the tissue salts magnesium and potassium phosphate; an herbal tablet with blood cleansing herbs such as echinacea, poke root, and red clover; vitamin B_5 for adrenal support; and a homeopathic kidney tonic.

Her esoteric treatment focused on the base and adrenal glands (adrenal triangle); throat chakra and the thyroid; the immune triangle (thymus and adrenal glands); lymphatic cleansing; the opening triangles involving the throat center and arms; and the grounding triangles involving the sacral and legs (sacral and hip minors, sacral and knee minors, sacral and feet minors). See appendix 1 for all triangles mentioned.

On her return visit, Grace reported slight improvement in her joints, fewer headaches, and an improvement in her intestinal function. The energy scan showed improvement in all areas except the lymph glands; they were probably dealing with a lot of stirred-up waste in her system. Her naturopathic and esoteric treatments were continued, and she made more improvements over the next few months. She had bad headaches from time to time, so magnesium orotate was given instead of the nerve tissue salt magnesium phosphate; this seemed to help. The joints continued to improve.

However, a new problem arose when she suffered kidney stones (base chakra problem). At this point, I introduced homeopathic kidney drops to help dissolve and remove the stones. She also had some medical treatment of a mechanical form by way of a stent (metal tube) to help pass the stones. I kept her on the kidney treatment for some time so that more stones did not form. From a naturopathic viewpoint, kidney stones are an example of calcium levels getting out of balance, as is so common with osteoarthritis. This stone formation was another indication that the energy in her system was congested and sluggish.

Not long before her retirement, Grace experienced a relapse with her joints, so we tried the popular new approach of glucosamine sulfate and chondroitin. This treatment helps to renew cartilage in the joints and restores the lubrication, but it takes a long time for the full effect to be noticed. Later, I had her try green mussel treatment. Clinical trials with a new type of extraction process from the mussel have shown positive results in Australian trials. Her basic remedies were continued for two years. Since her retirement, Grace has noticed that her health has generally improved and her joints are fairly good. She will probably need to continue the basic remedies for her joints and lymphatic system as a kind of health insurance.

Grace's case is most significant from the viewpoint of what can happen when the energy in the system becomes sluggish. She was not aware that her library work was having a slowing-down effect on the energies flowing through her skeletal system. She had to earn a living and library work was her training, and she belongs to a generation whose members do not usually change their occupation halfway through life. However, since her retirement, she has taken up working with immigrants to help them with their English. She finds this work very creative and has a new spring in her step. It is interesting that she is still working with language, but in a different way from the library work. Therefore, the throat chakra is still an important focus, but now the energies are flowing more adequately from the base center upwards. This is why her health has improved.

We can see how, in Grace's case, there is an interaction of chakra activity so that, while the base and throat chakras are significant, it is the base chakra and its relation to the adrenal glands that provides the basic energy for the system. The adrenal glands also have a significant role in immunity; although she was originally diagnosed with osteoarthritis, during the course of her treatment with me, further tests indicated it was rheumatoid, a more significant type of arthritis in terms of the immune system.

Of especial significance, in relation to her base chakra, was the tendency to form kidney stones, as the base chakra rules the kidneys. If the flow of energy is sluggish through the base center, then associated organs will be affected. With her new postretirement interests, her base chakra is much more energetic.

Sciatica and Disc Degeneration

One of the most common degenerative conditions involves the fourth and fifth lumbar vertebrae and the degeneration of the disc between them, and the resultant pressure on the sciatic nerve, which runs down the leg. The nerve becomes inflamed and swollen. Symptoms can involve lower back pain, groin pain, or discomfort down the leg. Osteopathic, chiropractic, and fascial therapy such as the Bowen technique will not restore the integrity of the vertebrae, but the realignment afforded by these treatments often takes the pressure off the nerve and it recovers. Sciatica involves a lumbar nerve as it leaves the spine, so it is related to the base chakra.

Particular minerals, combined with selected vitamins, can gradually restore the integrity of the discs, but these need to be taken for about two years. Calcium fluoride, in particular, is needed for the type of tissue in the discs, and is best combined with manganese, a zinc salt, vitamin E, and vitamin C.

Ivan, 51, had received naturopathic treatment over many years for persistent sinus problems and now revisited me after a business trip overseas. He was unable even to put on his shoes, due to acute sciatica that started before he left for overseas and steadily got worse during his three weeks away. He had seen chiropractors and physiotherapists for similar problems in the past and probably had some disc degeneration that would cause pressure on the sciatic nerve. After a Bowen treatment and taking extra magnesium and a homeopathic mixture (that included arnica for bruising, hypericum for nerve pain, comfrey for healing, and ferrum phosphate for inflammation), he was amazed at the resolution of the problem in a few days. As Ivan was also having regular treatment with me for sinus congestion, I was able to find out, over the next few months, that his back problem did not relapse.

During his Bowen treatments for the back, I included the main chakra balancing, vitality triangles, and grounding triangles for the pelvic and leg balancing.

As far as the base center goes, this is a very simple case, with no apparent significance at inner levels. But appearances can be deceptive, and I think there are some subtle implications with this recurrent problem. Ivan has a successful job and he and his wife lead the life of "high flyers," with frequent travel and a busy social life. They put off having children until their forties, but no pregnancy occurred. In keeping with sacral and base chakra weakness, Ivan was found to be deficient in healthy sperm. Overall, there was a certain lack of direction in his life, and this may be related to a poor flow of energy through his base center and spine. Resolution of his sinus congestion has been very slow, and I sometimes wondered whether this was related to the weak base center.

Ivan often quips that his life is not his own, and says that he is here for the purposes of others. This comment has an interesting connection to the will, the base center, and a lack of energy flowing from the base chakra upwards. When he first visited the clinic, many years before I began subtle healing on him, he was in the habit of only having naturopathic treatment, so the esoteric healing has not featured strongly in his case.

The next case history began the other way around, as the client came mainly for esoteric healing, rather than for naturopathic treatment.

Spinal Degeneration Case Study: David, 50, came to my clinic seeking help with back trouble after viewing a program on esoteric healing that I did on a community television channel. David, a physics schoolteacher, had suffered back problems for twenty years, despite consulting chiropractors and physiotherapists. X rays showed some degeneration of the spine, indicating the relationship of his problem with the base chakra. Other problems included bad hay fever after taking dairy products and a sluggish bowel. His iris indicated an overacid stomach; it was a moderately open iris structure that usually means basic minerals like calcium are out of balance, and it indicated bronchial weakness, another indication of poor calcium absorption.

I gave him the tissue salts sodium, magnesium, and calcium phosphate in colloidal form, liver and lymphatic toning drops, and I did Bowen Therapy, combined with esoteric healing. The energy scan revealed a weak base center and an energy disturbance in the lower spine. The esoteric healing, following the chakra balancing, included spinal work and the grounding triangles plus the vitality triangles, which involve two triangles that include the spine (lower pranic triangle and upper vitality triangle; see end of this chapter). On his second visit a week later, he reported some improvement. I added a disc support tablet that includes the above-mentioned salts, plus calcium fluoride, silica, manganese, and vitamins A and E; I also gave him anti-inflammatory herbs, and Bowen Therapy and esoteric healing were repeated.

After another three weeks, David reported less neck trouble, and his acidic stomach was improving. He continued to make gradual progress. A blood cleansing and liver mixture was then added to his program, because his bowel was still sluggish. By the end of five months of treatment, his back was better than it had been for many years.

David has a quiet personality and some people would see him as shy. He gives the impression, to some extent, of deficient strength, and this is probably related to the weakness in the base center. Any area devoid of sufficient energy for some years will eventually undergo organic changes; in this case, those changes involved degeneration of the discs. The sluggish bowel was probably also related to this lack of energy.

It is impossible in a few months of treatment to explore all the subjective causes of each ailment and, although he intended to come back for further treatment, David only took the minimum possible treatment, only until he felt his back was considerably improved.

Spinal Sinus

The next case is fairly rare, and I cannot remember treating any other spinal sinus case during my decades in practice. Again, anything connected with the spine will have a relationship with the base chakra.

Deborah, 38, arrived with a number of problems, including scalp eczema, fungal toe infections, heavy and long-lasting periods, and anxiety. Intermittently, she also had a sinus or cavity at the base of her spine, the most chronic of her physical conditions. I gave her a mixture with catmint, cat's claw, burdock, dandelion, and red clover for lymphatic cleansing, homeopathic liver and lymphatic toning drops, magnesium orotate for the anxiety, and homeopathic silica in a high potency for the sinus and for lymphatic drainage around the spine, scalp, and toes.

After a couple of months the spine trouble was much better, her periods were much lighter, and she felt more relaxed. The base chakra was more balanced. The eczema flared only periodically. Thuja 30 was added to her homeopathic drops for inherited tendencies towards the recurrent spinal sinus, and the subtle healing treatment was continued on each visit. In all, she had eight months of treatment and felt well enough in all respects to continue on the mixture and drops alone without seeing me any more.

I was surprised at how well this case resolved with the synthesis of inner and outer remedies. I find the high potency homeopathic remedies work better in combination with the esoteric healing. This is probably because the healing makes the psychic constitution more receptive to the effect of homeopathy. The high potencies have no physical molecules left, and work by resonance with the body and through the harmonics that reverberate in the energy field of the client. Deborah was receptive to the healing each month, and the synthesis of natural medicines and healing appeared to have resolved a condition that, in some cases, involves repeated surgery. Although the spinal sinus had been intermittent, a recent phone call to Deborah six months after the first draft indicated that it had not relapsed.

Rheumatoid Arthritis

Rheumatoid arthritis is an autoimmune disease, in which the body produces antibodies that attack the joints. Such antibodies can be found in the blood of persons with this disease. There is usually a familial incidence of this condition. The first joints most commonly affected are the small joints of the hands and feet; these take on a twisted appearance. Later, the spine and other joints can become affected. The disease is progressive, and the afflicted person can end up in a wheelchair and may possibly need extensive surgery for their joints. The most common medical treatment for the active state of this disease is cortisone, giving us the clue to the relationship: *the base center → adrenal glands → cortisone secretion.*

Two Rheumatoid Arthritis Case Studies: I have managed to keep Judith healthy over twenty years since her first visit. Judith is a teaching Sister who first visited me after a diagnosis of rheumatoid arthritis in 1981. She also had a history of thrombosis. Other symptoms included night sweats, irregular bowels, swollen ankles, and recurrent sore throats since the age of 18. At the time of her first visit, she was 34 years old. Her iris had a fairly fine structure, showing good vitality, but the presence of a particular type of brown spots indicated the inherited tendency for this condition. In the early 1980s, I was not doing the energy scan, but it was obvious from the history and symptoms and other observations how to proceed naturopathically. Over the last seven years or so, I have used esoteric healing on each of her visits.

Judith's first naturopathic prescription, in 1981, included herbs for the liver to improve the bowel action; anti-inflammatory herbs; vitamins B and C; homeopathic drops for balancing the endocrine glands; and the commonly used tissue salts for the nervous system, colloidal potassium and magnesium phosphate. On her return visit, she reported improvement in bowel regularity, cessation of night sweats, and less ankle swelling. She was still very tired, so a homeopathic nerve tonic was added. She continued to have bad sore throats for four months, and then only suffered them occasionally after I added an herbal mixture consisting of echinacea, phytolacca, violet leaves, burdock, and marshmallow. I gave her this mixture to work on the immune system and lymphatic glands.

Later, her esoteric healing recipe always included all the vitality triangles after the main chakra balancing; the adrenal triangle so that she could produce her own cortisone adequately; lymphatic drainage for the arms and legs; and the immune triangle (thymus and adrenal glands) because rheumatoid arthritis is an autoimmune problem in which antibodies produced by the blood destroy the body's own tissues. In this form of arthritis the joints are destroyed.

Judith has a very bright personality, and I could not discern what subjective factors may have been related to the arthritic problem, based on her appearance. However, she has always had a stressful job, and this can affect the base center and thus adrenal glands. From a naturopathic viewpoint, if the adrenal glands become deficient, then inflammation in the joints can easily occur.

From time to time, Judith gets a painful sore in the nose, so a high potency homeopathic remedy called Bacillinum is then used. It was interesting that many of her symptoms reminded me of the tubercular taint in the family tree and, in fact, I discovered that her mother had suffered tuberculosis. Bacillinum is an antitubercular miasmatic remedy. After some years of treatment, her homeopathic constitutional remedy became obvious *(Natrum Carbonicum)*, and this was given in a high potency with success. It sometimes takes a long time for the constitutional remedy to become obvious due to the effect of the complexity of modern living on a person.

Over the years the basic prescription for Judith has remained constant, with a few other remedies added or deleted. For many years, she had good results, in terms of energy, from royal jelly capsules, which are rich in B vitamins, which feed the adrenal glands. I also added vitamin E, for joint mobility, after she turned 40. Tablets containing bioflavanoids have also been used over the last few years for her veins and aching legs. Judith has stayed in excellent health, despite pressing professional obligations. She has been going through premenopausal symptoms lately, and she has used the extract from the wild yam to promote progesterone levels in her body, so as to keep the hormones balanced.

This case is a good one to illustrate how the synthesis of approaches can protect immunity, despite continuing stress in life. Judith does not wish to give up her contribution to the Catholic Church via her administrative career, and she wishes to continue a twice-monthly visit for health insurance purposes. The relationship between her rheumatoid condition and the base chakra is clear but, fortunately, she has not needed any cortisone and her joints have remained amazingly intact throughout the twenty years she has come to my clinic. The esoteric healing gave an added boost to her treatment, as she bounces back from most intermittent ailments, even though she is older.

Robyn, 44, represents another case of rheumatoid arthritis. She also has a positive attitude and has taken responsibility for helping this inherited tendency in a number of ways; her great aunt also suffered the problem. In Robyn's case, the trigger may have been hepatitis A and B. Before visiting me, she had taken some Chinese herbs, but still had sore hands and feet, with numbness in her hands and arms. Her iris revealed lots of acid in the connective tissues and moderate levels of toxins in the gastrointestinal tract. A scan of her energy field revealed that the liver was congested and her joints disturbed. In fact, the minor chakras in the hands and feet were closed, so without any energy flowing in those places, inflammation and pain could easily develop.

In relation to the base chakra, the most persistent problem with her health was not rheumatoid arthritis but proctitis, a persistent inflammation of the rectum, which is obviously in close proximity to the base chakra. Her proctitis was associated with a great urgency, at times, to reach a toilet for a bowel action and the passage of lots of mucus from the bowel. She had been given cortisone for this. Again, we see the relationship between the base chakra and its related endocrines, the adrenal glands. Cortisone is also the medical drug of choice for rheumatoid arthritis, so the challenge here is to regulate the base center and the adrenal glands so that she produces her own cortisone in sufficient quantities to resolve the proctitis and joint problems.

The esoteric healing included a focus on the base chakra, which was somewhat depleted of energy, the vitality triangles, lymphatic drainage to help clear the accumulation of mucus, and work on the thymus gland to improve immunity. The chest triangle of force was included to strengthen the thymus gland—i.e., throat minor and breast minors. Special attention was placed on the minor chakras of hands and feet by doing the opening triangles for the throat and hands and grounding triangles for the sacral center and feet. The healing was continued at each visit, and as the hand and feet chakras stayed open, her pain in these areas diminished.

Her first naturopathic prescription included St. Mary's thistle herb for her liver, plus homeopathic liver and lymphatic drops, vitamin C (2 g daily), anti-inflammatory herbs, and the tissue salts potassium and magnesium phosphate for the nervous system. On her return visit, Robyn said her joints had improved but she still had some numbness in the hands. So I added colloidal calcium phosphate to her prescription and chondrosamine sulfate as further support for the joints. Vitamin B complex was included for energy. At this stage, the proctitis was not too active.

At her third visit, Robyn reported that her joints were much better. She was having deep tissue work, and this helped greatly with the swelling between the fingers and, intermittently, with the numbness. By the fourth visit, the numbness was further reduced and she was delighted to report that the rheumatoid antibodies had been reduced to zero. The rheumatoid specialist was very surprised and told Robyn to go on with what she was doing. She also undertook to do work at the psychological level.

Later she went overseas for a short trip and, as happens so often with long-distance flying, her autoimmune condition flared and I found the thymus gland to be disturbed on her return. It took several weeks for her health to return to the previous level of improvement. The proctitis is still not fully resolved, but has improved.

In summary, this case has a lot of interesting factors. There is the inherited tendency from her aunt for rheumatoid arthritis. Inherited tendencies often stay dormant if the lifestyle is good. In this case, an unhygienic immunization in Asia resulted in hepatitis B. Although this event happened many years before the autoimmune disease manifested, it probably affected the immune system and the inherited predisposition eventually emerged. In addition, there was an accumulation of acid waste in the tissues that probably coincided with the time when the liver was below par; thus the joints became inflamed. The accumulation of waste resulted in excess mucus in the system that tended to affect any area of weakness; it manifested in rectal inflammation.

From a naturopathic viewpoint we have a classic retracing from the chronic stage (arthritic joints) to the sub-acute stage (mucus excretion). This is why the proctitis will be the last problem to resolve.

From the esoteric perspective, the main issue was keeping the base chakra balanced and energized. There may be sensitive issues from Robyn's past that relate to the weakness of this chakra that have then influenced the adrenal glands. There was also a weakness of the thymus gland that, at times, got triggered by, for instance, long flights; this pointed to the need for continuing the attention on the chest triangle of force at each healing session.

As the thymus gland is related to the heart, there may also be old issues affecting this chakra. In keeping with my esoteric approach, I do not delve into the past if the client is making good progress; I prefer to take their mind off past problems by providing the inner alignment that allows healing energies to flow from their soul.

Clients repeatedly report that the result of the healing alignment during the session is profound relaxation, a sense of peace, and serenity. From my perspective, this is their response to the alignment created between the soul of the healer and themselves.

We move now to a case that had no direct, outer connection with the skeletal system, but is, rather, a simple case of adrenal exhaustion following shock.

Adrenal Exhaustion Case Study: Joan had been involved in a serious train accident thirty years earlier. She had suffered exhaustion ever since, and was now in her late fifties.

When doing the etheric scan, I found that her base chakra was depleted and that the energy in both adrenal glands was disturbed. The healing consisted of chakra balancing and vitality triangles. The latter were of particular importance in this case, as the lower pranic triangle and upper vitality triangle involve the base chakra, which conditions the adrenal glands. In addition, the adrenal triangle was visualized and the adrenal glands themselves traced in light. After the healing, I gave Joan homeopathic drops specifically for the adrenal glands, vitamin B complex, and the tissue salts magnesium and potassium phosphate for the nervous system. She could hardly believe the difference in her energy after a few weeks. Many months later, I was pleased to find that she had not relapsed.

This case illustrates the fact that some chakra disturbances will manifest only in a disturbance of the associated gland (in this case the adrenal glands), rather than spreading further to the associated organs and tissues. We also see the profound effect of an old shock over many years and the need, therefore, to take a careful client history. Again, we see the value of treating the person from both an inner and outer perspective, as the physical remedies toned the adrenal glands

> *As the thymus gland is related to the heart, there may also be old issues affecting this chakra. In keeping with my esoteric approach, I do not delve into the past if the client is making good progress; I prefer to take their mind off past problems by providing the inner alignment that allows healing energies to flow from their soul.*

concurrently with the restoring of the underlying energies in her etheric field.

As the repository of the will to survive and to be, the base chakra houses a lot of energy in health. In most chronic disease, in the face of fear or exhaustion, these basic energies are depleted. We have considered here some case histories featuring ailments of the organs or tissues conditioned by the base center including osteo- and rheumatoid arthritis, lower back pain, sciatica, kidney stones, a calcified shoulder, and adrenal exhaustion.

The minerals needed for the skeleton (mentioned earlier) show the base center in its connection with the Earth and with the basic energies that this chakra involves. Often, towards the end of the healing process, I visualize a line connecting the minor center below the solar plexus of the client with the Earth, if they need grounding and energizing with the energy taken in by the base center.

Healing Practice with the Base Chakra and the Vitality Triangles

You can now start to practice triangles that will help to energize your body. These energies involve the base chakra, adrenal minors, spleen chakra, sacral chakra, and throat chakra. Study the diagrams of these vitality triangles and the adrenal triangle before and during the exercise. Here is how to do them:

1. Align as previously described. Place your hands on the client's shoulders and imagine linking up with your own soul, the client's soul, and the source of all healing, and ask that healing take place according to the plan of the soul.

2. Visualize the healer's flow of energy by imagining the following alignment: soul, heart, head, and hands.

3. When you sense that the energies are flowing, move to the left-hand side of the client and kneel or sit so that you can comfortably have your hands on either side of their body. From this point on, you do not need to physically touch the client.

4. Balance all the chakras up the spine, as described earlier, by placing the right hand behind the spine of the client and the left
hand in front. Sense the impact of the energies on the hands and
move them gently in and out, in an accordion fashion, until the
flow of energies seems balanced between your hands.

5. Balance the chakras in the order of solar plexus, base, sacral,
heart, and throat. During this process, there is no need to have
your hands close to the client's body. It is best to have them as
far away as possible, because it seems easier to assess the energies
in this way and it is less disturbing to the client.

6. Stand a few feet behind the client and imagine connecting your
brow chakra to their base center and also connect the hand
chakras, in thought, with the adrenal minors. As before, do not
be too concerned about whether you are visualizing the minor
chakras in exactly the right place above the kidneys. Remember
that energy follows thought, and after connecting the three
points, visualize lines of light between the three points.

7. Wait a few moments until you have a sense of energy flowing
freely through this triangle. This triangle is called the **adrenal
triangle** (see figure 13).

8. Then do the **spleen triangle,** which is one of the vitality triangles which bring in energy to the body. Stand a few feet in front
of the client. Connect your brow chakra with the solar plexus,
and imagine connecting one hand chakra with the spleen chakra
and one with the spleen organ itself.

9. Visualize lines of light connecting these three points and wait a few
moments until you sense that the energy is flowing (see figure 14).

10. Now move to the **lower vitality triangle,** which involves the
base, sacral, and spleen chakras. Connect your brow chakra with
the base chakra, one hand chakra with the sacral chakra and the
other with the spleen.

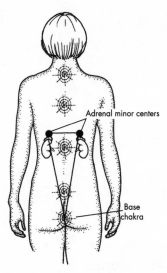

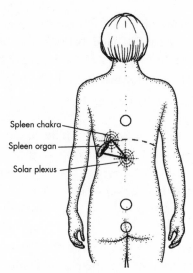

FIGURE 13: THE ADRENAL TRIANGLE. The adrenal triangle links the base center with the adrenal minor centers situated near the adrenal glands on top of the kidneys. When vitalized, this triangle brings energy into the body via the base center, adrenal glands, and kidneys.

FIGURE 14: THE SPLEEN TRIANGLE. The spleen triangle brings energy into the body via the spleen chakra, spleen organ, and solar plexus chakra.

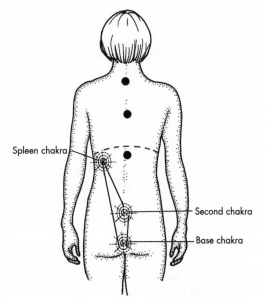

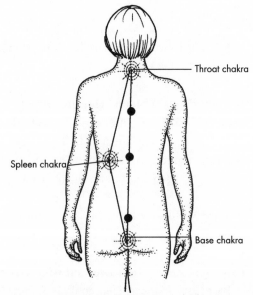

FIGURE 15: THE LOWER VITALITY TRIANGLE. The lower vitality triangle links the base chakra, spleen center, and sacral chakra. It is an important triangle for bringing energy into the physical body.

FIGURE 16: THE LOWER PRANIC TRIANGLE. The lower pranic triangle is another triangle that brings energy into the body via the base, spleen, and throat chakras.

11. Connect the three points with light and wait a few minutes until you sense that energy is flowing freely (see figure 15).

12. Make the **lower pranic triangle** by moving your right hand from the spleen and up to the throat chakra. The brow chakra stays connected with the base and the left hand with the sacral center. The three points of the lower pranic triangle are the base, sacral, and throat chakras (see figure 16).

13. As before, hold these points for a few moments and sense the energy flow.

14. Close the aura of the client by using your hands or imagination to make the shape of an oval aura around the client, from the feet upwards, using a gentle sweeping motion. Imagine gently withdrawing the healing energy back through the hands to your soul, so as to break the connection with the client, now that the healing is completed.

15. Visualize closing up your own aura, in whatever way seems best, or imagine the same movement on yourself as you used on the client.

9 The Sacral Center and Reproduction Disorders

Treating disturbances involving the reproductive system form a large part of my practice. I find this area interesting, because there is such complexity and interaction between the inner and outer factors, this being a main theme in this book. Infertility, ovarian cysts, menstrual irregularities, endometriosis, sexual problems like impotence, menopause, prostatic enlargement, and cancer of various parts of the reproductive tract all feature as physical disorders associated with a disturbance of the sacral chakra.

The subjective factors associated with the sacral center involve food, sex, and comforts. Our use of money to supply these needs is therefore involved. You may remember that sacral chakra consciousness, apart from food, sex, and comforts, is associated with the creative use of money; in this sense, balance in the sacral center enables us to ground our schemes. If we consider the topics featured in the popular media, books, magazines, and television programs, there is a big emphasis on food, sex, and home comforts, indicating the interest of the general public in these areas.

A large section of humanity is learning to understand sexuality in a far more open manner and to transmute sexual energy into creativity, related to the throat chakra. This process can only take place after our sexuality is acknowledged and owned, rather than suppressed. So there are, temporarily, many energy problems and physical disorders associated with the glands related to these chakras, the ovaries and thyroid. Therefore as with the other chakras, we cannot separate sacral chakra disorders from the influence of other chakras, such as the solar plexus or in particular, the higher counterpart of the sacral center, the throat chakra.

The sacral chakra conditions its associated glands, the ovaries in the female and testes in the male, plus all the associated tissues, including the uterus, fallopian tubes, bladder, and the prostate gland in the male. Therefore, congestion or contraction of the sacral center or enlargement, as compared with the other centers, will tend to cause disturbances in the associated organs of the body.

For instance, I have noted that, in most overweight women, the base and sacral centers are much larger than the other chakras. This enlargement may be associated with overeating or with other sacral issues, such as intimate relationships or the need for comfort. As we know, comfort eating often takes place when a person is emotionally disturbed; it is, therefore, a blend of solar plexus desires and the need for comfort (sacral) issues.

In most people, there is a big interaction between the solar plexus and sacral chakra, because the desires associated with the solar plexus stimulate the sacral center. This can cause overactivity of the sacral center, followed by its depletion. Physical ailments can occur at either stage, contraction or enlargement.

Inherited predispositions feature more strongly with the sacral chakra than with other chakras, because of the common occurrences of venereal taints in one's family tree. I am thinking, in particular, of female problems, such as cystic ovaries or fibroids. Exacerbation of inherited problems results from using drugs, such as the contraceptive pill, and from a poor diet. If we add the stressful living of the twenty-first century, we have a mix of factors that makes for plenty of reproductive ailments. The disorders that we will explore in this chapter include menstrual irregularities, cystic ovaries, infertility, menopause, cystitis, and prostatic cancer. At the end of the chapter, you will find healing exercises for the sacral center and reproductive organs.

Ovarian and Gonadal Imbalance

Probably the most common endocrine disturbance in my female patients is related to their ovaries. In particular, from age thirty onwards, the two hormones produced by the ovaries get easily out of balance in Western women. The estrogen becomes dominant over the progesterone. Symptoms of this include weight gain, particularly of the hips and legs, fibrous lumps in the breast, heavy and painful periods, migraines associated with ovulation or menstruation, ovarian cysts, lack of libido, spotting between periods, endometriosis, and mood swings. You probably know many women who have some or all of these symptoms.

Many of these problems have greatly increased since 1980. Why? The causes are multiple. Since 1960, a large percentage of women have used the contraceptive pill and that can cause an imbalance in these hormones. The liver metabolizes progesterone more quickly than estrogen, so it is easy to see that a person using the contraceptive pill over one or two decades could gradually put on weight from an excess of unmetabolized estrogen in the tissues. It appears that Western women are more prone than women in Asia to this problem, perhaps because they take estrogen supplements to prevent conception and after menopause. Other causes include the stress of twenty-first century living and our typically poor eating habits. On this point, there has been considerable controversy about whether Asian women have greater hormonal balance because they take phyto-estrogens in the form of soy products.

As the ovaries slow down towards menopause, estrogen tends to become dominant, although levels of both ovarian hormones diminish greatly at this age. Both are excreted in much lower levels, yet estrogen is often dominant over progesterone, in terms of levels. As John Lee, M.D., explains in his excellent book *What Your Doctor May Not Tell You About Menopause*,[42] most menopausal symptoms are caused by estrogen dominance. These symptoms include hot flushes, depressions, fluid accumulation, weight gain, spotting between periods, fibrous breast lumps, and mood swings.

Many of these symptoms are similar to what younger women experience, except for the hot flushes. Dr. Lee explains how using the progesterone precursor extracted from wild yam can protect against breast and ovarian cancer. As mentioned earlier, the cream is used as a topical application on the thighs, breasts, and stomach.

The following is a typical case among dozens of women I have treated who had this hormonal problem of excess estrogen compared to progesterone.

Hormonal Imbalance Case Study: Chris, 46, originally visited me with a history of heavy and painful periods, flatulence, and moderately high cholesterol. She also had recurrent upper respiratory infections each autumn. Her iris indicated a build up of acid in her tissues, but her inherited constitution appeared good, as judged from the regularity of the iris fibers. Her diet may have contributed to her acidity, as she always used white bread; otherwise, her diet was good.

Chris's first prescription was mainly directed to improving her metabolism through the digestion, cleansing the acid from her tissues, and balancing her nervous system. She was given an herbal digestive mixture with meadowsweet, gentian, angelica, dandelion, cranesbill, and marshmallow root; homeopathic liver and lymphatic cleansing drops; and magnesium and potassium phosphate in colloidal form for her nervous system. After one month, she reported that the flatulence had improved, her period was much better, and she had lost some weight.

The prescription was repeated, and I did not see her for a year, by which time she was closer to menopause. She now had very sore breasts and was carrying a lot of fluid each month from ovulation onwards. This indicated that the drop in her progesterone each month was too great to prevent the symptoms previously described. In other words, after a certain age, progesterone drops off more quickly than estrogen, and this is the cause of the estrogen dominance. When I checked her energy field, the ovaries were disturbed and the sacral chakra ruling the ovaries was larger than the other chakras. This is a very common finding with overweight women who also have ovarian imbalance.

The mineral salts for the nervous system were repeated, and Chris was given vitamin C (2 g daily) for general detoxification and the progesterone cream to apply to the skin from the day of ovulation to the start of the period. Chris was already taking herbs for sinus and digestion matters. I conducted the esoteric healing for the energy field each month, and used the sacral and grounding triangles (see end of chapter) after the chakra balancing, lymphatic cleansing, and vitality triangles.

After one month, she reported that her breast pain had improved and her energy was better. An energy scan revealed that her chakras were now balanced and the ovaries no longer disturbed. A further month of treatment resulted in no clotting or pain with her menstruation and no breast swelling, and she had plenty of energy. Her improvements continued.

I include this case here, because it is typical of so many I see. Invariably, in cases of ovarian imbalance, the sacral chakra will initially be much larger and more dominant in terms of energy than the other chakras. The inner or subjective factor may be an inability for some women to use the sacral energy creatively. So this means that some women have not learned to use the throat center to draw the energy up from the sacral energy for more mental creativity. This is especially important at the time of menopause, when the ovaries slow down. Creative meditation is useful here.

Apart from the external factor of excess estrogen coming from the contraceptive pill and disturbing the balance, Chris needs to make sure she is creatively fulfilled in some way, to prevent excess energy building up in the sacral center. The fact that Chris improved so quickly indicates that the imbalance was mainly caused by outer factors. This impression concurs with the fact that she gives the impression of being an active and creative woman.

In menopausal cases, the progesterone cream may be continued for several years, or even permanently, as a health insurance against breast or ovarian cancer. Be clear that this is *not* synthetic progesterone, as used in the contraceptive pill or hormone replacement therapy. The dosage of the cream is generally tapered down after all symptoms have abated for some months. Another point to note is that many of the wild yam creams on the market are fairly useless. The cream needs to be a concentrated extract from the yam. It is usually combined, for successful use, with other herbs such as chaste tree, so do your research carefully before you purchase a progesterone cream.

Polycystic Ovaries

Another common problem associated with estrogen dominance is polycystic ovaries, which means the woman has a number of ovarian cysts. There is often an inherited predisposition for the problem, and the condition is often associated with infertility. It appears to be related to an imbalance of hormones that can be corrected naturopathically.

First Polycystic Ovaries Case Study: Pam's was a typical case of this condition. She visited me at age 26. Her menstrual period occurred only once every three months. Blood tests revealed that she was not ovulating, and that this was caused by the cystic state of her ovaries. She was overweight, listless, anxious, and suffered heartburn after eating particular foods, although her diet was fairly good.

Pam's mother had a hysterectomy at age 31, a fact that may indicate the inherited tendency to her problem with the ovaries. She had been taking the contraceptive pill steadily from ages 14–22, with only short breaks. On top of a predisposition to cystic ovaries this was certainly a prescription for disaster, in terms of hormonal imbalance, and would be responsible for her early weight gain.

The main signs of imbalance indicated in the iris were increased acidity in the tissues and an imbalance of the autonomic nervous system, which is closely related to hormone activity. My energy scan revealed a disturbance in the ovaries and sacral chakra enlargement. It also indicated that the sacral center was out of balance and that the other chakras were enlarged. The ovaries and lymphatic system in the pelvis showed energy disturbances. The esoteric healing included the chakra balancing and vitality triangles, plus lymphatic drainage in the pelvic area, and the grounding triangles to take of excess energy from the blockage in the sacral area (see appendix 1).

I gave Pam natural progesterone cream to apply topically throughout the month; homeopathic liver and lymphatic cleansing drops including Thuja, in the 30th potency, to remove the inherited tendency towards cysts; calcium phosphate in colloidal form for the ovarian cysts; potassium and magnesium phosphate in colloidal mineral form for balancing the autonomic nervous system; and vitamin C for detoxification and the B complex for energy.

After one month, Pam reported that she had a period that was less heavy and painful, that her energy was improved, and she had suffered a cold. I explained that this was a common occurrence in the first two months of treatment as part of the cleansing process. Her heartburn was still intermittent and she had started to see a psychologist for her anxiety. During the healing, I found that her chakras had become more balanced and the ovaries were no longer showing an energy disturbance. At her next visit, Pam reported that she had more energy, but had suffered a very heavy period. I advised increasing the dosage of progesterone.

The basic remedies were continued, and Pam took a large supply of her supplements with her for a trip lasting some months. In her most recent report, she said her periods were fairly regular and that she was feeling well.

Pam's case resolved quickly, due to her positive attitude and generally creative stance towards life. She and her partner planned the trip around Australia as a creative interlude in their lives and were prepared to face the challenge of possible difficulties finding work on their return. Her decision to travel for the purpose of having a complete break from busy working lives was, perhaps, a factor correcting any subjective aspects of her sacral problem. The esoteric healing corrected the underlying disturbance in Pam's ovaries.

On the physical side, despite the inherited factor predisposing her ovaries to be cystic, they responded well to the physical and esoteric treatment and Pam's cycle returned to a normal rhythm after a few months of treatment.

Although I have treated numerous cases of polycystic ovaries, there are individual differences between cases, and each person, therefore, receives individual treatment. Some remedies, such as the colloidal calcium phosphate, are typically given to strengthen either ovaries or kidneys that manifest cysts. Sometimes, as in the following case, the calcium is combined with colloidal sodium phosphate to keep the calcium in solution in order to avoid or accommodate digestive imbalance.

Second Polycystic Ovaries Case Study: Rebecca, 32, had a complicated case of polycystic ovaries and suffered an excess of testosterone. This male hormone had changed her hairline to a masculine distribution pattern, and her ovulation was suppressed. She had not had a period for three months at her first visit. Other problems included a history of asthma from the age of seven, for which she was taking preventive medication. In her midtwenties, she had suffered sub-acute thyroiditis, which means an inflammatory process in the thyroid. She had been on the contraceptive pill earlier in her life and had developed high blood pressure as a result; she was now taking medication for this problem. There was a history of diabetes in her family.

Rebecca's iris indicated complications. It showed brown spots of a type that we often associate with inherited miasms (mentioned earlier), and this indicated the tendency, in her case, to ovarian trouble and hormonal imbalance. The iris showed there was a moderate level of toxins in the gastrointestinal tract. The scan of her etheric body indicated problems with the pituitary gland, ovaries, adrenal glands, and most of the digestive organs. The chakras were imbalanced accordingly; there was an excess of energy in the sacral center and base center, and a deficiency in the throat center.

After the basic chakra balancing and vitality triangles were given, the esoteric healing included the adrenal triangle to balance the adrenal glands, the sacral triangle to balance the ovaries, and the endocrine pentagon to balance the pituitary, adrenal glands, and ovaries together. I also did the lymphatic drainage technique; as her digestive organs were disturbed, I added the digestive triangles (see appendix 1).

Rebecca's first prescription included a mineral tablet in colloidal form, containing sodium phosphate and calcium phosphate for the cystic ovaries; vitamin C (2 g daily); homeopathic liver and lymphatic cleansing drops to help her digestion and start the cleansing process; homeopathic drops to balance all the endocrine glands; and a natural progesterone-promoting cream to use three out of four weeks each month. The subtle healing was included each time she visited.

At her first return visit, Rebecca said she had suffered some disturbance during the second week of treatment, but had noticed her hairline problem was improving and that she had managed to reduce her cortisone dose for asthma. After another month the dosage was again halved, but she still had not had a period.

After three months of treatment, Rebecca started to have periods, although there was a space of 37 days between each. Her hairline became almost normal for a female, and blood tests revealed that her testosterone levels had been reduced and, concurrently, her periods had become more normally spaced. It is common for testosterone levels to be raised in cases of cystic ovaries. I noted that her energy scan showed no disturbances; in fact, I noted that, prior to this point, the disturbances in the energy field underlying the glands cleared up very quickly. However, it takes time for changes to filter down to the physical cells.

So she did not get a period for two months after I noticed the energy had corrected itself in the glands. This underscores the value of using *both* the inner healing and outer naturopathic treatment. If I had just done the healing on her energy field she would not have had a period, because the body needed the basic minerals and homeopathic remedies to correct the biochemistry at the physical level.

Rebecca's hormonal levels became completely normal after nine months of treatment and she came completely off steroid treatment for her asthma. Her menstrual cycle was then regulated to a 33-day cycle, which continued over the next few months. It is likely that it may normalize further.

The high testosterone levels and their resolution made this an interesting case. All women secrete some testosterone from their adrenal glands, and, for some reason, it is often higher than normal in cases of polycystic ovaries. It was ten times higher than normal in Rebecca. The extra energy found in her base center would account for extra stimulation to the adrenal glands, leading to increased testosterone production.

Further interesting factors in this case were the imbalance of several chakras (base, sacral, and brow) and their associated endocrine glands. The blood pressure problem was probably related to the excess of adrenal activity, and perhaps her asthma medication of cortisone for many years added to her circulatory problem. Rebecca is now off all asthma and blood pressure medications and no longer has recurrent and severe viruses. While she does not yet have a normal 28-day cycle, she is at least having periods within a six-week time span. Her esoteric healing now is like a maintenance treatment, and I rarely find energy disturbances in her chakras or organs.

Infertility

Infertility is a major modern problem in Western countries, and often results from the hormonal imbalances previously described. The xenoestrogens (foreign chemicals that mimic estrogen in the body) from the environment have unbalanced the ratio between progesterone and estrogen. When hormonal imbalances are combined with mineral deficiencies and inherited tendencies, we often have ovarian malfunction. Almost without exception, when I do an energy scan on an infertile woman, the energy underlying one or both ovaries is disturbed.

Infertility Case Study: Katrina, 36, had been trying to conceive for fourteen months, yet all the medical tests had proved negative, meaning that no reason for infertility could be found. Her iris revealed chronic nerve rings and moderate toxins in the gastro-intestinal tract. If you look at an iris with a flashlight, you will see it is composed of fine fibers that radiate out from the pupil. Chronic nerve rings mean that the iris shows deep circular furrows in its radial fibers, and this indicates a long-standing deficiency of minerals in the nervous system, usually potassium phosphate. Katrina suffered from tension headaches, as predicted by the nerve rings. Periodically, she developed oral herpes (cold sores). Her diet was good and she had just given up drinking coffee.

Although the medical tests proved negative, I found, prior to doing esoteric healing, that the sacral center was deficient in energy, and one ovary had disturbed energy. After the main chakra balancing and the usual vitality treatment, the sacral triangle, endocrine pentagon, and grounding triangle were visualized on Katrina.

In Katrina's first month of naturopathic treatment, she took colloidal calcium and magnesium phosphate to tone her nervous system and, therefore, to help her headaches; the antioxidant vitamins C and E; liver and lymphatic toning drops plus homeopathic drops for balancing the endocrine glands; and wild yam extract to apply as a cream on the skin from ovulation to the onset of her period to balance the hormones. The esoteric healing was undertaken to correct the energy imbalance underlying the ovaries.

Infertility is a major modern problem in Western countries, and often results from hormonal imbalances. When hormonal imbalances are combined with mineral deficiencies and inherited tendencies, we often have ovarian malfunction. Almost without exception, when I do an energy scan on an infertile woman, the energy underlying one or both ovaries is disturbed.

On her return visit, Katrina reported having suffered a heavy cold and a cold sore. The mucus elimination that happens in a cold often manifests in the first month of treatment and indicates that the vitality of the body is improving such that mucus elimination is now possible. I gave her homeopathic *Natrum Muriaticum* to take weekly, in a high dose, for the cold sore tendency.

At the second visit, Katrina reported that she was already five weeks pregnant, which means she was pregnant towards the end of the first month of treatment. She and her partner were delighted. She was to continue treatment with me throughout the pregnancy, to ensure the health of the baby and herself, especially during the first trimester, to prevent any miscarriage because of her age. A woman in her mid-thirties is more likely to miscarry, because the hormones may not be flowing consistently from the ovaries as in a younger woman. Once the placenta takes over the role of producing the hormones for the pregnancy after the first trimester, there is far less likelihood of miscarriage.

Katrina is one of many cases of apparent infertility that I have treated. It is an especially joyful task to help a couple produce a child. During the esoteric healing sessions for the purpose of encouraging pregnancy, I attempt to become aware of a soul that may be intending to incarnate with the parents I am treating. Sometimes, I am aware of a vibration of love that I interpret as an unborn entity wishing to take birth through the mother. I had this experience with Katrina. Her case seemed otherwise devoid of any complications from the physical or subjective side.

If we provide the right functional and biochemical parameters for the mother then, provided it is the destiny for the mother to conceive a child, the event can happen. In Katrina's case, the energy problem involving the ovaries appeared to correct itself easily with the esoteric healing, while the natural medicines balanced the biochemistry. This is a good example of synthesis in healing in practice.

Endometriosis

Endometriosis is, in part, a hormonal condition, and from a naturopathic point of view, it is caused by an excess of estrogen. Often this accumulates as a result of using the contraceptive pill, consuming excess estrogens in foods such as force-fed chickens, and through a drop in natural progesterone levels that often starts after Western women reach thirty. There is also, from a homeopathic point of view, an inherited factor that comes from familial tendencies previously mentioned.

In endometriosis, we see the development of extra uterine tissue anywhere in the abdominal cavity, such as on the ovaries, fallopian tubes, uterus, or bowel. This tissue is under hormonal control, which means that it has a monthly cycle and it can bleed into the abdominal cavity, sometimes at the time of ovulation and during menstruation. It produces a fair amount of pain when this happens. Multiple cysts can be found in the ovaries and uterus; adhesions and scarring within the pelvic cavity are common in this condition. Currently, diagnosis is usually made by laparoscopy, and treatment involves medical lasers.

Endometriosis Case Study: Melissa, 35, visited me ten years ago, with endometriosis and candidiasis (a yeast overgrowth). She had a baby aged twelve months, but at the time of her visit, Melissa had apparent infertility that she was hoping to resolve with natural therapies. She had been diagnosed with two cysts on the right ovary and one on the left. Her iris was finely structured, with moderate irregularity of the autonomic nervous ring, indicating a hormonal imbalance.

An energy scan revealed a disturbance underlying the ovaries and uterus, and a disturbance in the lymphatic glands in the groin. I had not started doing esoteric healing on every case at this point, although I was regularly doing the energy scans for diagnostic and prescribing purposes.

Melissa's first month's treatment included colloidal calcium phosphate and potassium chloride for the cystic tendency; a zinc salt for resolving the pelvic adhesions; an herbal mixture containing blue cohosh, echinacea, motherwort, and meadowsweet for cleansing the lymphatic system and for hormonal balancing; and homeopathic drops for balancing the endocrine glands and for further lymphatic cleansing.

After one month of treatment, she had less pain and flooding with her period, and the candidiasis had disappeared. By the second month of treatment, Melissa was pregnant and later delivered a healthy girl after a very easy labor. Her candidiasis returned while she was pregnant, but disappeared after the birth. A Candida infection (candidiasis is an infection by *Candida albicans*) is often stimulated by the extra hormones generated during pregnancy. An energy scan, after several months treatment, indicated that there was now a healthy flow of energy through the ovaries, uterus, and lymphatic glands.

Further consideration may be necessary as to the effect of female hormonal imbalance derived from their mothers. Melissa brought her daughter, now seven, for advice about pubic hair already developing at this young age and about large fleshy warts on her left leg. The warts are an inherited tendency, for which homeopathic Thuja may be the remedy. The early appearance of pubic hair is a tendency becoming quite common in young girls who have been subjected to abnormal hormonal input from their mother and environment. I gave the daughter basic cleansing and hormonal balancing treatment, plus the Thuja drops for the warts, and today she is doing well.

Prostate Tumor Case Study: The most common reproductive problem for men over fifty, apart from impotency, is either benign or malignant growths of the prostate. Benign hyperplasia, as it is called, can move in a malignant direction. It has been found that 50% of men over fifty years old have some enlargement of the prostate. From a naturopathic viewpoint, this is often associated with a zinc deficiency and, therefore, from a zinc deficient diet.[43]

From an esoteric perspective, the sacral chakra is involved and is usually found to be congested, together with energy disturbances underlying the prostate gland. Looking at the psychology aspect, it is open to conjecture as to whether there are problems and frustrations in the sex life of many of this large group of men. Often, men in this age group complain of impotence, and I suspect this is partly hormonal, partly psychological, and partly due to general lack of energy. It is interesting that many men in this age group would have been smokers in the middle of the twentieth century, before smoking incidence dropped as a result of education about its harmful effects on the circulatory system. Included in possible circulatory problems of male smokers is the loss of elasticity in the delicate capillaries, which govern the erectile strength of the penis.

The prostate gland surrounds the urethra and, therefore, one of the main symptoms suffered by men with enlarged prostate is difficulty in passing urine and increased desire to urinate. They especially notice this during the night, when they have to keep getting up to empty their bladder. Natural treatment is very successful for many enlarged prostate cases.

Gavin, 60, came to our clinic with diagnosis of a growth in the left side of the prostate. The prostate specific antigen (PSA) levels indicated possible malignancy. He had suffered difficulty in passing urine for seven years, and recently had a urinary tract infection. From a psychological viewpoint, he was a bit depressed that his job in a timber mill meant separation from his wife, except at the weekend. You will remember that the sacral center relates to the handling of money, and

Gavin was disturbed that his poor financial situation meant that his wife had to work in town and he had to work in the countryside.

His iris revealed a moderate acid build-up in the connective tissue, accompanied by a lack of minerals, lymphatic congestion, and irregularity in the function of the autonomic nervous system. His diet was reasonably good in terms of protein, vegetables, and grains, but it was lacking in fruit. He consumed from a half to one bottle of wine daily, which is too much for the health of the prostate gland.

From an esoteric perspective, his sacral chakra was congested and the energy underlying the prostate gland disturbed, together with disturbances in the lymphatic system. My impression was that there could well be a malignant change in the prostate.

Gavin's naturopathic prescription included vitamin C (1 g, twice daily) for the infection and immunity; the colloidal minerals iron phosphate and potassium chloride for inflammation and fibrous tissue; zinc chelate equivalent to 15 mg daily; and an herbal tablet with andrographis, echinacea, and olive leaf for the current infection. He was also given specific homeopathic drops for the prostate and its tumor formation.

His esoteric treatment included general chakra balancing, the vitality triangles, sacral triangle, and lymphatic drainage, plus the immune triangle. Gavin had a very positive attitude and felt very peaceful during the healing. After one month, he returned and reported passing urine more easily and that his urinary infection had gone, according to his doctor. He decided not to go ahead with surgery for the time being. Vitamin E was added to his program as another important antioxidant. A live blood analysis by another therapist suggested that he was suffering from candidiasis, so I gave him lactobacillus, bifidus, and bulgaris bacteria in capsule form to rectify that situation.

His subtle healing regimen was continued, and I found that his energy field had remained in balance at the second and third visits. He then had another PSA test for prostate cancer, and it was found to be almost normal. His surgeon suggested there was no point in even doing a biopsy of the prostate. Gavin has maintained his good health and has had no surgery.

This case suggests that the prostate was enlarged for some years before the swelling and the move towards a malignant condition.

There were sacral problems involving money issues, and the separation from his wife each week was experienced as depressing. Gavin had the courage to try alternative medicine before he went ahead with surgery. I was a bit concerned at this decision, and in no way encouraged him to cancel the surgery, but the synthesis of treatment appears to have completely resolved his problem.

The following case was not nearly so favorable in its outcome, but it indicates what happens when the inner conflicts are not resolved, despite both naturopathic and esoteric treatment.

Prostate Cancer Case Study: John, 60, had been coming to my clinic for many years for exhaustion. He had a high-pressure job that entailed a lot of car travel each week for a government department. A main problem was that he could not organize his life to have suitable time for his personal life. After a traumatic divorce following a second marriage, he developed rampant prostate cancer. He chose to have invasive radiation treatment, which left him with intermittent hemorrhages from the rectum.

Despite comprehensive naturopathic treatment, esoteric healings, and radiation, the cancer did not clear, according to the usual blood test for prostate evaluation. Finally, he was given an estrogen implant, after it was discovered that the cancer had spread to the right hip. At this stage, I introduced bovine tracheal cartilage, because it has the effect of preventing the division of cancer cells.

John's was an interesting case, because the cancer was so clearly related to his inability to work on the causes leading to ill health, despite many suggestions and discussions. The basic cause for his ill health appeared to be that he was a workaholic who would not make space for his own needs. It would be interesting to know whether John's two failed marriages were related to lifestyle issues. We had many discussions as to how he could rearrange his life, but with each different job, he appeared to have the same problem—an inability to say no. In terms of the sacral center, money was a major problem, as his second marriage breakup resulted in a very poor financial situation. It was this problem that goaded him to overwork. He was interested in doing a workshop on esoteric healing before his cancer was diagnosed, but later, despite nine months of sick leave on pay, he never actually managed to do self-help studies, meditation, or anything creative to resolve his lifestyle problems.

One of his main activities during this period was to fulfill the demands of an ailing ninety-four-year-old mother, who expected him to visit her daily, and to whom he felt responsible, although she was in good full-time care. He carried out all instructions for his naturopathic medication exactly, consulted two other healers at my suggestion, but, from my viewpoint, did not explore the underlying causes for his cancer.

John always experienced benefit, in terms of increased energy, from his healing sessions. Apart from the usual regimen of chakra and vitality triangles, I added lymphatic drainage, immune system, sacral, and grounding triangles, and aspirant's triangle. John took bovine tracheal cartilage and used the hormone implant for a few months, after which his PSA evaluation was nearly normal. He left his high-pressure job with all the traveling, and, with his good track record for project managing, obtained a job as a manager of building projects at a girl's school. However, despite his aim to only work part time, he soon found himself as pressured with work as ever. Further, he created a small business for himself and once again was traveling all over the state.

John has had extensive naturopathic treatment for well over a decade, but he remained still dependent on a therapist and did not provide space for his own needs. John had a temporary improvement with both energy and antibody levels for cancer following an estrogen implant. However, as he got into the same problem of overwork with his building supervision at the girl's school, his health deteriorated very quickly and the stress caused serious problems with his liver. At this time, he admitted to me that I had been right all along and he should have listened to suggestions about changing his lifestyle. But it was too late—his liver seemed unable to metabolize the high levels of estrogen from the implant, and he suffered constant nausea and exhaustion. He died a couple of weeks following hospitalization for liver failure.

This case illustrates how no amount of holistic treatment can help if the client is unable to follow a suitable lifestyle and remove stresses that threaten his immunity and well-being. At the time when John first went to the girl's school, his health was starting to improve and, for the first time in years, he had more energy. But he quickly fell into the same trap as in his previous job and worked seven days a week. His tendency to be optimistic was misplaced, and two weeks before he died, he was telling me how he would change his life when he went home from hospital. So the other main point to make here is that we need to be realistic about our health situation. Holistic therapy means that a person needs to be sufficiently integrated to recognize warning signs in time to act appropriately.

Bladder Infection Case Study: The kidneys and ureters chiefly relate to the base chakra, but the conditions associated with the sacral center will also include any conditions associated with the bladder.

Nancy had suffered bladder infections for five years before I started treating her. The infections were severe enough for her to pass blood. Nancy's is an unusual case, because her bladder was highly sensitive to environmental changes involving the weather. She had severe pain in the bladder and pelvis if exposed even to the cold temperature of an air-conditioned supermarket in summer. She was also suffering menopausal symptoms, with hot flushes plus a Candida infection. Her iris revealed a weakness in the kidney and bladder area, a general build-up of lymphatic congestion and acidity throughout the body, and moderate toxic accumulation in the bowel.

From an esoteric viewpoint, both her base and sacral center were low in energy, and, at the first scan, her uterus, ovaries, and bladder showed energy disturbances. The sacral center disturbance was, in her case, related to both the bladder and menopausal disturbances. Her esoteric healing included the chakra balancing, vitality triangles, and sacral triangle; I made an additional triangle with the bladder and kidneys. The lymphatic drainage was included for cleansing the pelvic area and assisting immunity. Nancy always seemed depressed to me, so, at the end of the healing session, I always included the "chest triangle of force": throat minor and breast minor chakras to bring in love energy associated with the heart; I also used one of the triangles for spiritual development—solar plexus, heart, and brow, also known as the "clearing triangle" (see appendix 1).

Nancy's naturopathic treatment initially included an herbal mixture for immunity against the bladder infection and included olive, pau d'arco, motherwort, and astragalus. She was already taking the antioxidant vitamins C and E, plus vitamin B complex, and the minerals magnesium and calcium. I added the mineral tissue salt sodium phosphate, and, after a few months of only moderate improvement, I started to think in terms of deep-acting constitutional homeopathic remedies. I came to the conclusion that she needed *Natrum Phosphoricum* in a very high potency. She took one drop of this every second week and, after three months, we stretched it out to once monthly. Nancy started to turn the corner after the inclusion of this homeopathic remedy, such that, after years of bladder trouble, she has remained in stable health for eighteen months now.

This case illustrates the success of using a synthesis of remedies and approaches. The basic vitamins, minerals, and herbs were not working until we added the homeopathic remedy in the M potency. This is such a high dilution that, if you were to write out its full equation, it would have 1,000 zeros! Such a potency penetrates right into the psyche and reverberates into the emotional life. Combining subtle healing with this deep-acting remedy allows it to work more easily and fully. In other words, the healing smoothes away the blocks in the psyche that might slow down or prevent the full action of the homeopathic remedy.

Summary of Sacral Chakra Disorders: The sacral center has been discussed in terms of disorders related to the reproductive system and, to some extent, in relation to the related psychological issues. There can be inherited predispositions as, for instance, in some cases, involving cystic ovaries. There are also factors that are sometimes detrimental relating to substances we take into our bodies, such as the contraceptive pill, hormone replacement therapy, and food. Successful holistic treatment occurs when there is a *synthesis* of outer and inner treatments. As with the other categories of disorders, we cannot separate the sacral chakra off from the others in a particular ailment. There may be influences from disturbances of the solar plexus and throat chakras, in particular, impinging on any reproductive disorder.

Healing Practice for the Sacral Chakra and Reproductive System

Although I will focus on the sacral triangle, grounding triangles, and the endocrine pentagon after this chapter, remember that when practicing on a client, first balance all the chakras, then do the vitality triangle practice after the base center to bring in energy. So now, having learned the vitality triangles, the sequence for healing is alignment, balance the chakras, vitality triangles, then addressing the particular problem in question; in this case, the reproductive organs.

1. Align as previously described. Place your hands on the client's shoulders and imagine linking up with your own soul, the client's soul, and the source of all healing and ask that healing take place according to the plan of the soul.

2. Visualize the healer's flow of energy by imagining the following alignment: soul, heart, head, and hands.

3. When you sense that the energies are flowing, move to the left-hand side of the client and kneel or sit so that you can comfortably have your hands either side of their body. From this point on, you do not physically need to touch the client.

4. Balance all the chakras up the spine, as described earlier, by placing your right hand behind the spine of the client and your left hand in front. Sense the impact of the energies on the hands, and move them gently in and out, in an accordion fashion, until the flow of energies seems balanced between your two hands.

5. Balance the chakras in the order of solar plexus, base, sacral, heart, and throat. During this process, there is no need to have your hands close to their body. It is best to have them as far away as possible, because it seems to be easier to assess the energies in this way and is less disturbing to the client.

6. Move a few feet in front of the client to do the **sacral triangle.** Visualize connecting the brow chakra to the sacral center, which is situated just above the pubic bone.

7. Imagine connecting the left hand chakra to the right ovary minor chakra of the client (on your left) and the right hand to their left ovary minor chakra (see figure 17). Imagine lines of light between these three points.

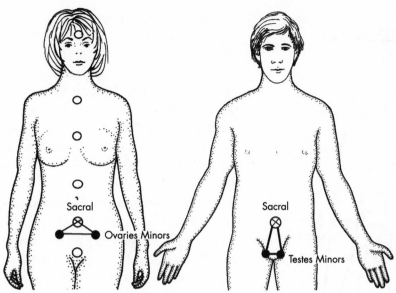

FIGURE 17: THE SACRAL TRIANGLES. The sacral triangle involves the sacral center and the ovaries or testes, and is vitalized for the purpose of regulating the sex hormones.

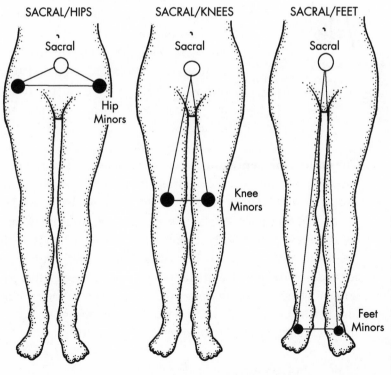

FIGURE 18: THE GROUNDING TRIANGLES. The grounding triangles bring the energies down through the legs and feet, so that excess energy is removed and the individual is literally more grounded in all their activities. It also removes congestion in the pelvis and energy blocks in the hips and legs.

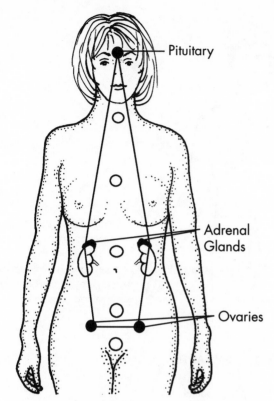

Pituitary

Adrenal Glands

Ovaries

FIGURE 19: THE ENDOCRINE PENTAGON. A pentagon means that we are visualizing five points, in this case, the pituitary gland, adrenal glands, and testes or ovaries for the purpose of balancing the hormones.

8. As with every triangle, hold the three points until you sense the energy flowing. You can make a triangle, in imagination, between the ovaries themselves and the uterus and imagine tracing these organs in light with your imagination. In the case of males, you will be making the triangle between the sacral center and the minors associated with the testes.

9. To do the **grounding triangles,** keep your brow chakra focused on the sacral center and visualize triangles between the sacral center and hip minors, then sacral center and knee minors and, finally, sacral center and foot minors (see figure 18). Wait while doing each triangle until the energy seems to be flowing. The purpose of these triangles is to ground energy that has been accumulating excessively, not only in the sacral center, but also in the whole body or to psychologically "ground" someone who needs to be more practical by developing the ability to materialize their ideals.

10. The **endocrine pentagon** is used for balancing the hormones in cases of premenstrual tension, irregular periods, post menopause problems, and infertility (see figure 19). There are five points here, as the name suggests, so place, in imagination, your brow center on the brow center of the client, and place your hands so that one hand chakra points to the adrenal gland and ovary on the left side of the client and the other hand addresses the other adrenal gland and ovary. Remember that energy follows thought and it is mainly our thought in the healing process that counts in these relationships between the healer and the client.

11. Close as in the previous exercises.

10 The Heart Chakra, Circulatory System, and Immunity

The circulatory system comprises the heart, arteries, arterioles, veins, and capillaries. The heart is the one organ that almost everyone knows, in terms of position and basic function. The associated endocrine gland is the thymus, situated just above the heart in the chest cavity. This gland produces hormones, which are intimately associated with immunity, as they enable the T lymphocytes, made in the bone marrow, to mature. There is a close relationship between physical immunity and the correct functioning of the heart chakra. If the heart chakra is affected by shock, depression, or grief, the thymus gland and immunity can suffer.

In a psychological sense, the heart chakra is associated with unconditional love, and the healthy functioning of the heart chakra gives psychic immunity. This means that energies flowing freely through the heart give us immunity to the negative emotions and thoughts of other people. It has been found that physical immunity becomes depressed, as measured by the groups of white blood cells associated with immunity, when we become depressed or angry.[44]

In relation to the energy fields underlying the physical organs, the magnetic field emitted by the heart is 5,000 times greater than the brain and is, by far, the most powerful energy field emitted by the body. This pulsating magnetic field can be measured by a Super Quantum Interference Device (SQUID).[45] This field is closely related to the functioning of the heart chakra and has been measured in relation to healing. So from an esoteric healing viewpoint and the naturopathic perspective, the heart and its associated chakra are important to the health of the thymus gland.

We can consider the physical heart as an organ that nourishes all the cells throughout the body via the blood and as an organ associated with the strongest flow of energy in the body. This energy is related to the "vitality" always mentioned by natural therapists; it is the energy that conditions our immunity and is involved in healing.

It will help you understand how esoteric healing works if you consider the research of William Tiller, professor of material sciences at Stanford University, in California. He found that when a person concentrates on their heart and thinks of another person with appreciation, love, and tolerance, a coherency of heart, brain, and respiration is established between the two people. This coherency has been found to enhance health and well-being, as measured by various psychological and physical scales.[46] This underscores the alignment process for our healing protocol, whereby we bring energies from the heart to the hands. It seems that, if the healer is in a healthy state, the energies from their heart can produce well-being in the client.

From a naturopathic perspective, the promotion or lowering of vitality can now be seen to be intimately related to the magnetic field of the heart. The heartbeat is obviously related to the magnetic field. Perhaps this is why cardiologist Irving Dardik, M.D., found that the heart rhythm must stay flexible for health. In all chronic disease, Dr. Dardik found a rigid pattern in the heartbeat, whereas, in health, there are minute variations between heartbeats.[47] Perhaps the need for a slight heart rate variability corresponds to the thymus gland and immune system adapting to various needs in our lives.

In this chapter, we will include case histories for heart and circulatory problems, such as high and low blood pressure. Disorders with lowered immunity, such as glandular fever, are featured, plus several cases of thymus gland disturbance related to autoimmune disorders, including multiple sclerosis and lupus. I have included chronic fatigue syndrome (CFS) in this chapter, because it is also related to low immunity. In addition, I discuss the effect of immunization on the immune system and asthma cases that seem to be triggered with the immunization regimen applied to young babies and children.

We will start with the circulatory problem of high blood pressure, and then move to the more complicated disorders involving the immune system.

High Blood Pressure

High blood pressure is one of the more common conditions I face daily in my consulting practice. The majority of cases are, in my view, caused by deep nervous stress although the client is usually unaware of this tension in their body. The problem is intimately related to the sympathetic nervous system and to excess activity of the adrenal glands and its related chakra, the base center. This causes a dilation of an energy center, known in Chinese medicine as *Meng Mein*, situated behind the spine, at the level of the navel.

The Meng Mein is not exactly a minor center, in the usual sense of the word; it can be considered more of an accumulation of energy that a person with high blood pressure suffers, in relation to their adrenal glands. It has a reflex action on the heart, causing excessive contraction and a lessening of relaxation between beats during diastole (the name given to the pressure within the heart when it is at rest). If the heart remains stressed and partially contracted when it is supposed to be at rest, this is a dangerous condition for the heart over a period of time. This is why physicians are especially concerned when the lower reading of the blood pressure (systole over diastole) is raised, because this reading relates to diastole. Formerly, the major medical concern related to the possibility of the person having a stroke, but more recently, the problem of the heart being unable to relax has been highlighted as a major cause of heart failure.

There are, of course, other reasons for high blood pressure, such as kidney disease and blocked arteries, but the majority of cases appear to be related to stress. I find clients suffering high blood pressure to be therapy resistant, so I think we need to look at the heart and circulation from a broader viewpoint.

High Blood Pressure Case History: Leonie is a middle-aged mother with seven children. She has visited me, on and off, over several decades for health problems in herself or her children. Most of these problems have related to the lymphatic system, and have manifested in nearly all the family members as eczema. Recently, she came with high blood pressure, a condition that had not responded to medical treatment. She wished to try another approach.

Her iris diagnosis indicated considerable accumulation of toxins in her tissues, and lymphatic congestion showed up as small yellowish clouds around the edge of the iris. She also had a number of brown spots, like freckles, on the iris; these are called psoric spots, and indicate the tendency to eczema in her children.

The energy scan revealed an imbalance in the chakras, chiefly with too much energy flowing through the base center and congestion in the heart chakra. The excess from the base center would stimulate the adrenal glands to secrete too much adrenalin, and the extra adrenalin would increase the blood pressure, which could cause severe strain on the heart. This overactivity of the base center can come from stress and tension in the body, caused by any stressful condition in life; in the case of Leonie, the stress began with her heart, in a psychological sense, due to her concern about particular members of her large family.

I gave Leonie magnesium orotate, homeopathic liver and lymphatic toning drops twice daily, and an herbal sedative containing passaflora, vervain, skullcap, and hops. I balanced all her chakras and applied the vitality triangle, adrenal triangle, high blood pressure triangle (brow, heart, and spleen), followed by the chest triangle of force, to give strength to her heart (see exercise at the end of this chapter).

To ease her stress, I taught Leonie a simple exercise that would balance that part of the nervous system related to those activities of the body not usually under the control of the will: heart beat, blood pressure, and digestion. This part is called the autonomic nervous system and consists of the sympathetic part, which is related to the adrenal glands, and the parasympathetic part, related to the vagus nerve. The sympathetic part has become dominant in our twenty-first-century stressful living, increasing heart beat, blood pressure, and breathing rates.

In other words, the sympathetic nervous system, when stimulated, causes the fight-or-flight syndrome. To reduce the effect of this aggressive process, we need to stimulate the parasympathetic part, in particular, the vagus nerve. We can do this by relaxation or meditation exercises so that the whole system can become serene again.[48]

Here is an exercise for reducing blood pressure:

1. Find a quiet place where you will not be interrupted for ten minutes.

2. Play peaceful music in the background.

3. Focus on your breathing by counting on each out breath. Count one on the first out breath, two on the second, three on the third, and then go back to one. Repeat this for about ten minutes.

4. Do not deliberately breathe slowly, but notice how the breathing and heartbeat slow down. This is a good exercise to do whenever tension is present, such as in the dentist's chair or when waiting in a line.

I teach this breathing exercise to all my blood pressure patients, but most of them do not carry it out morning and night for ten minutes as suggested. However, Leonie has been a good case, and has persevered such that her blood pressure condition has completely resolved without drugs. I never suddenly stop blood pressure medication with the patient, but usually combine it with natural therapies for some months before suggesting a gradual reduction.

When Leonie returned after a month, her blood pressure had dropped ten points. After a further month, it dropped another ten points, and then after three months it was normal and it has stayed there. She has been doing the relaxing exercise regularly and also uses it to get to sleep.

The case of Leonie illustrates the synthesis needed in diagnosis and treatment. Although the first observation related to the excess energy flowing through the base center, the underlying stress related to her being the mother and prime caretaker of a large family; it was, therefore, related to her "heart" concerns. It was not sufficient to give her the physical remedies and to do the chakra balancing, for she needed to have some means of preventing the stress from developing. The daily relaxation exercise with the breathing provided that means.

I am finding an increasing number of persons consulting me to resolve blood pressure problems. I attribute this to the pace of twenty-first-century living, plus the strain that some people place themselves under. Some personality types push themselves to unreasonable limits to achieve what other individuals perceive as unnecessary for the satisfaction of personal ambitions. We are all different in personality characteristics, and life would be boring otherwise. But some people seem to go to extremes, and need to be encouraged to become more creative and involved with life and others for their own health.

Second Blood Pressure Case Study: Glenda, 52, has used natural therapies for many years, and was introduced to them when she became our clinic bookkeeper several decades ago. She revisited me recently with a high blood pressure reading of 140/100, chest pains, and shortness of breath. The diastolic blood pressure of 100 is too high for the heart when it is supposed to be at rest, and this fact probably related to her chest pains.

Her cholesterol levels were 6.5, instead of the recommended 4.5, and she had been admitted to hospital for investigation before visiting me. Nothing was found, except a deficiency of oxygen in her blood. She was also light-headed and suffered from nose bleeds. Her iris revealed an accumulation of toxins in the gastrointestinal tract, and her diet was only fair, marked by the consumption of eight cups of coffee daily. She was not on any pharmaceutical medication.

Glenda's naturopathic treatment consisted of magnesium orotate twice daily to relax the nervous and circulatory system; an herbal sedative containing passaflora, valerian, scullcap and hops; liver and lymphatic toning drops; and drops for bringing oxygen and hydrogen into the tissues. I gave her flaxseed oil daily to reduce the cholesterol, and she promised to reduce her coffee intake.

Her energy scan revealed congested energy in the heart area, with an accompanying blockage in the heart chakra. This blockage manifested as a lack of free-flowing energy through the heart chakra; it was possibly related to the chest pains. The esoteric healing treatment consisted of the general chakra balancing, vitality triangle, and then specific work on the heart and circulation. This included the blood pressure triangle (brow, heart, and spleen), circulation technique for gently wafting the blood around chest and head, and the vagus triangle for relaxing the nervous system (brow, alta major, and spleen).

After one month of treatment, Glenda's blood pressure was restored to normal and she was feeling much better. She took one month more of treatment, and did not need to return. A year later, she was still in excellent health.

Although Glenda improved in health, I would have preferred that she continue treatment for a longer period, as she tends to push herself very hard at work; it is likely that her stress levels will rise and cause further problems. It would have been very helpful, in her case, to practice the stress reduction exercise.

Third Blood Pressure Case Study: Father John, 63, is a Catholic priest under enormous pressure with his workload. He has many duties apart from conducting church services, baptisms, weddings, and funerals. His other duties include pastoral care for a large number of parishioners, plus various church functions at different times of the year. When he first visited me, he was on blood pressure medication, and came for a general checkup. His iris revealed a good constitution and other moderate health problems, including a few twinges in the knees, dating from old sporting injuries, a tendency to sinus congestion, and a concern about his digestion. His blood pressure while on the medication was 146/90. He was in the habit of doing lots of exercise in the form of running each morning.

His first prescription consisted of magnesium orotate for relaxing the arterial system and nerves; dandelion for the liver, plus echinacea and other herbs for the lymphatic system; vitamin C for his immunity; liver and lymphatic drops for digestion and cleansing; colloidal iron phosphate and potassium chloride as a mineral combination for reducing the inflammation and exudation from the sinuses. His esoteric healing included the blood pressure triangle of brow chakra, heart, and spleen.

I was a bit nervous, at first, to suggest esoteric healing to a priest, but Father John accepted this procedure as a valuable part of the treatment. I find that, after he has been busy with his work, the energy center associated with the adrenal glands (the Meng Mein) behind the waist is enlarged. There have been times when he was stressed and his heart organ showed disturbed energy, with accompanying enlargement of the heart chakra compared to the other chakras.

After two months on this regimen, all conditions had improved and his blood pressure had dropped to 126/85. As this level was consistent for many months, we decided to try curtailing his drugs and found his blood pressure remained within safe limits. Later, I added vitamin E (250 mg daily) as a circulatory aid and antioxidant. The use of vitamin E for people with high blood pressure tendencies needs to be considered carefully, as this vitamin stimulates the heart muscle;

it is safe to use in low dosages, such as prescribed here. Due to his high-pressure work, Father John has chosen to continue with the supplements and esoteric healing as health insurance.

Low Blood Pressure

Low blood pressure is not harmful, unless it is so low that the person is in danger of fainting. Most low blood pressure is due to a lack of energy through the base chakra and lack of energy in the adrenal glands, which, in turn, reduces the amount of circulating adrenalin. This indirectly affects the heart energy.

Low Blood Pressure Case Study: Denise, 45, has worked as a school counselor and teacher, so she has a fairly stressful job. She requested treatment for light-headedness and vague headaches that were probably related to her low blood pressure which was 96/60. This meant that the systolic blood pressure was under 100, which usually gives tiredness and, in some people, a fainting tendency. She also had aches and pains in the elbows, knees, and finger joints.

Low blood pressure is not harmful, unless it is so low that the person is in danger of fainting. Most low blood pressure is due to a lack of energy through the base chakra and lack of energy in the adrenal glands, which, in turn, reduces the amount of circulating adrenalin. This indirectly affects the heart energy.

Her physical remedies included a B complex for energy and a component of the B group (vitamin B_5) to stimulate the adrenal glands, which are intimately related to blood pressure. Vitamin E was given to increase blood pressure by stimulating the heart action, and colloidal potassium phosphate was added to stimulate nerve function. She was also given the liver and lymph-toning homeopathic drops.

An energy scan on Denise indicated a deficiency of energy in all the chakras and this related to her general tiredness. As with all clients, I found that, after the healing, the energy flow of the chakras was restored. However, without the physical remedies, the chakras may have lost energy during the month. There is a two-way flow, involving the energy field—from the remedies to the energy field and from the psyche to the energy body. So again, a synthesis of healing approaches was necessary in this case.

Denise was a woman who drove her body too hard, but instead

of this raising the blood pressure, it had the opposite effect, producing exhaustion and low blood pressure. This difference in possible outcomes probably relates to the inherent strength of the adrenal glands and heart. Again, we cannot easily separate one chakra and accompanying glands from the others.

Over the first few months of treatment, her improvement fluctuated, but her joints improved and her headaches diminished; the light-headedness and dizziness fluctuated from month to month. I added another homeopathic remedy for dizziness and an herbal tranquillizer containing valerian, passaflora, gentian, and hops; and a rheumatic herbal tablet for her joints, as these relapsed in the winter. Her blood pressure came up to between 100/75 and 105/75 and, although she had some relapses with periods of vertigo, she remained well thereafter.

Denise elected to continue her treatment as a form of health insurance for many years, reducing her visits to once every three months. As the years passed, her nervous system became very stable and she managed to get through periods of stress at school without any relapses. She learned how to manage viral infections with large amounts of echinacea, colloidal iron phosphate, potassium chloride, and vitamin C.

From an esoteric viewpoint, circulatory problems are an important indication about the flow of our life energy throughout our constitution and into the environment. Although all the chakras are involved, the heart chakra is that basic part of our esoteric constitution associated with circulation of both energy and blood. The base center, in relation to the adrenal glands, is an important subsidiary consideration. If we experience blocks or frustrations to our life force, it can become dammed up, and eventually result in an "explosion" known as a stroke. This is a simplistic explanation and needs to conjoin with an understanding of the arterial condition, and inherited and lifestyle factors. In addition, our emotional states have a profound effect on the heart, while relaxation exercises can have a health-giving effect on the heart and circulation.

The Thymus Gland and Immunity

We now move from conditions directly related to the heart and circulation to conditions with the thymus gland and immunity. At the beginning of this chapter, the relationship between the heart chakra and its associated gland, the thymus, was mentioned. The thymus gland is intimately related to our immunity. Not only does it develop several categories of white blood cells known as T lymphocytes, but it also stimulates antibody production in other white blood cells. The interactions between helper cells, suppressor cells, killer cells, and antibody production is complex, and new facts about immunity are constantly being discovered.

When white blood cells circulating in the blood and lymphatic system encounter an antigen (foreign protein) in the form of, for instance, a virus, they form antibodies. When the body next encounters the same virus, the antibodies lock on to the foreign protein and destroy it. The production of antibodies by the plasma cells is called humoral immunity. Other white cells have the job of engulfing and digesting the unwanted particles, a process called phagocytosis. Evidence suggests that the current childhood immunization process will trigger an existing predisposition of a Type 1 sensitivity in some children and cause eczema or asthma. The use of vitamin C before and after immunization will minimize this effect.

We all know people who have a very good lifestyle, including exercise and good diet, yet who suffer chronic asthma, hay fever, or mucus discharges of various kinds. From a naturopathic and homeopathic viewpoint, these are individuals from a family usually conditioned by ancestors who suffered tuberculosis or gonorrhea. We are not talking about an active form of the disease, but an inherited *tendency* for certain ailments. Sometimes when I question a person about their family tree, they have heard of a grandmother who had tuberculosis. However, the problem may go back to further generations, about which there is no known history. In the case of gonorrhea or syphilis (the other venereal taint affecting family trees), families are not likely to shout these histories from the housetops.

The gonorrheal taint has a tendency to provide the basis for widespread disorders such as uterine fibroids, cystic ovarian and kidney disease, asthma, herpes, and any mucus and purulent discharges from the reproductive organs or respiratory system. Included here are conditions like acute and chronic bronchitis, bronchiectasis, ear and eye infections, vaginal discharges, and cystitis. There may also be triggering factors to these conditions, such as smoking, poor diet with deficiency of vitamins and minerals, nervous exhaustion, and environmental pollution. However, behind most persistent immune problems will be the inherited *predispositions* or chronic miasms. Homeopathy is able to resolve many of these inherited predispositions that affect the immune system.

From my perspective, there are, at times, inner factors predisposing one towards infection. The thymus gland and one's immunity can be badly affected by negative emotions, particularly grief, as mentioned earlier in relation to the heart chakra. However, in many cases, the outer factors predominate, such as poor nutrition, environmental toxins, use of pharmaceutical and recreational drugs, epidemics, and a poor constitution (as previously discussed under the area of chronic miasms). In other cases, there is a combination of both inner and outer factors.

We will start our examples of immune deficiency with a simple case that had no complicating psychological factors, but needed only natural therapies to support the immune function. However, subtle healing was still included, because it enhances the immune system and the effect of remedies prescribed.

The following cases are all related to the need for increased immunity. They move from infections to the more chronic cases involving autoimmune disease, where specific antibodies attack the body's own tissues. I find this latter category interesting in relation to the heart chakra. Is it possible that, if we do not love ourselves sufficiently, a self-destructive process can take place in the body? Perhaps. But we also know that there is an inherited factor in autoimmune disease, such as rheumatoid arthritis, and in Hashimoto's disease, which effects the thyroid.

Infections—A Case Study of Boils: Dale, 21, is a kitchen hand by trade. He visited me with an unpleasant neck infection of two years duration. The problem started with an infected cyst on the back of his neck that was lanced by a doctor. It developed into a very resistant infection that manifested as repeated boils on the neck that were resistant to all antibiotics. Dale had a good diet, consuming lots of fruit, wholemeal bread, salads, and vegetables. According to iris diagnosis, his constitution was good. As he was a worker in a restaurant kitchen, it was obviously important to resolve his problem as soon as possible. From an esoteric perspective, I found, from my scan of his etheric body, that the lymphatic system contained chaotic energies, so I directed the esoteric healing accordingly.

I gave Dale 4 g of vitamin C per day; 15 mg of elemental zinc twice daily; a mineral combination of the tissue salts for the three stages of inflammation with colloidal iron phosphate, potassium chloride, and calcium sulfate, three times daily; and an immune-stimulating herbal mixture containing equal parts of catmint, *Echinacea purpurae*, cat's claw, yellow dock, and burdock, 10 ml twice daily. (When I talk about three stages of inflammation, from a naturopathic view, I mean initial inflammation, clear serous discharge, and infection, as in pus.)

The etheric energy scan noted congestion in the lymphatic system. Esoteric healing included chakra balancing, the vitality triangle, in particular, the lymphatic cleansing for the lymph glands around the neck area, and the immune triangle of thymus and adrenal glands.

After two weeks on this regimen, the infection started to come under control; by one month, it seemed to have cleared completely. Then Dale became slack with the treatment and the infection started to recur. He resumed treatment, and was later able to stop treatment after five months without relapse.

This uncomplicated case is one we could place in the category of an infection from an outside source, which may have been a cross-infection that occurred in the doctor's office in a vulnerable area of the body. Dale's general health was good and his diet was excellent, so he made an uncomplicated recovery, as soon as he was given the right remedies to help his body fight an infection that had all the signs of drug-resistant staphylococcus.

However, it was obvious from his temporary relapse that he needed to be consistent with the treatment for some months. The emphasis here was not on any subjective factors in the psyche of Dale, although the esoteric healing helped the physical remedies along by correcting the underlying energies of the lymphatic system.

Asthma

In Australia, one-in-four children suffer from asthma, so this is one of the most common conditions that relates to a disturbance in the immune system.[49] It is also related to mineral deficiencies involving calcium; to congestion in the lymphatic system from poor diet and metabolism; and to predispositions in the family tree to tuberculosis. This condition leads to poor assimilation of calcium, so that the tissues of the lungs and bronchial system are weak. The family tree may also feature gonorrhea, which accounts for the mucus tendency in the bronchial system of asthmatics. We could say that inherited predispositions can affect the immune system, when combined with environmental factors.

Asthma is related to one type of allergic reaction called Type 1 sensitivity. A person of this type reacts very quickly to certain foreign proteins with swelling and secretion. Examples of such proteins may be grass, a particular pollen or virus, and certain phenolic substances in foods. In its extreme form, this type of sensitivity to foreign proteins can trigger anaphylactic shock, as occurs very occasionally after a bee or wasp sting. In this type of reaction, there is massive swelling that often cuts off airways, such that immediate medical intervention is necessary.

However, the average asthma sufferer is not so severely affected, and mainly suffers from wheezing and mucus production that, to various degrees, restrict their airways temporarily. Foreign protein, in the form of viral material, can cause asthma following an infection, and this is a very common problem in children who have an asthma tendency. Natural therapies are able to regulate the immune system, so that children have reduced and milder infections with no associated asthma. The following case is typical of this.

Asthma Case Study: Simeon was first brought to me after his first asthma attack at age three. He had been subject to a lot of respiratory viruses. His mother had wisely removed cow's milk from his diet, which otherwise included a lot of fruit, vegetables, whole grain cereals, and breads. His iris indicated considerable deficiency of minerals; this was indicated by the structure of the fibers in the top layer of the iris, which, in this case, were open and dispersed. There was some stress in his family life, because his single mother had to work full time and Simeon was in childcare.

His first prescription included vitamin C, colloidal calcium phosphate to strengthen the chest area, echinacea tincture for his immune system, and liver and lymphatic toning homeopathic drops, combined with Thuja in a medium potency. Thuja resolves the gonorrheal family miasm, which may go back five generations or so.

These remedies were continued for many months, and Simeon made consistent improvement throughout this time. He relapsed for a short time a few months into the treatment after eating chocolate Easter eggs. A homeopathic phenolic compound was then introduced to resolve any of his allergies to food substances.

An etheric scan of Simeon revealed disturbance to the lymphatic system, and the energy flowing through the throat, heart, and solar plexus was jerky. With young children, I often do a subtle form of esoteric healing, whereby I only visualize the balancing of the chakras and the triangles. In this case, the various triangles for the chest were visualized without using my hands at all. These triangles included the lung triangle (throat and lung minors, diaphragm triangle), vagus minor and diaphragm minors, and chest triangle of force (throat minor and breast minors; see appendix 1). This extra subtle healing seems to work suitably, as children are very sensitive to flows of energy. I recommend practicing the healing this way for some time before doing it on others.

From time to time, Simeon had some nervous instability and fears after starting school, so we added magnesium phosphate to his calcium salt. Magnesium has a stabilizing effect on the nervous system in this form. Exposure to chlorine from swimming pools tended to make his eyes very red, and he had a mild virus from time to time, but no associated asthma.

After his immune system was stabilized, the echinacea was removed from his prescription, and his minerals were gradually reduced to a maintenance dose as a means of health insurance. I continued him on the vitamin C, for the same reason. He also was given flaxseed oil, as a dietary supplement for his tendency to have dry skin; this oil is rich in unsaturated oils and the omega 3 group, and also helps the immune system. Simeon is now six years old and has not suffered asthma for three years. He is very well also in other respects, namely, his general nervous and muscular strength.

It is a thrill to see undersized and immune deficient children begin to flourish and stabilize with the help of a few natural substances. However, understanding and compliance on the part of the mother is very important in this process. I find that most children under fourteen years do not tend to take much responsibility for their health and are dependent on the enthusiasm of the mother to devise ways for them to take their medication on a regular basis. When you think of the alternative of repeated antibiotics or cortisone-based "puffers" for many years, this is not a big sacrifice for a mother to make. Usually, I find young children are able to take their drops in a small amount of water or juice; the minerals can be chewed, as they are without flavor.

For children who have deficiencies in a number of vitamins and minerals, perhaps as a result of very poor eating practices, manufacturers of vitamins and minerals have produced pleasant-tasting multivitamin tablets that can be combined with other specific treatments for their disorders.

Herpes Simplex (Cold Sores)

One of the most common conditions that people suffer when their immune system is run down is herpes or cold sores, which usually develop on the mouth or in the nose, often after an upper respiratory infection. The problem can be associated with swollen lymphatic glands; as they are the "policemen" of the body, we are reminded of the need for a clean lymphatic system for healthy immunity. It seems likely that the manifestation of herpes simplex is the result of weakness in the immune system. I have found that this condition responds rapidly to natural remedies, and hardly ever recurs after six months or so of treatment.

Herpes Case Study: Heather, 43, is a teacher who was exhausted when she first came for a consultation. She had injured her rib cage through heavy lifting, and then manifested a fever. She had suffered severe cold sores for years, so that her specialist thought it might be connective tissue disease associated with an autoimmune process. Her iris showed a moderate level of toxins in the body, a depleted nervous system and markings that indicated an inherited tendency towards skin problems. Her diet was moderately good, but stodgy, as she ate lots of pasta. Due to her poor immunity, as indicated by the cold sores, and for cleansing purposes, I advised her to take two glasses of raw juice daily, consisting of equal parts of carrot, apple, celery, and a smaller amount of raw beet, on an empty stomach.

The supplements prescribed were an herbal mixture that included catmint, cat's claw, burdock, and astragalus for immunity, plus the herb motherwort as a nerve tonic. Further support for the nervous system was provided by colloidal magnesium and potassium phosphate; she was already taking vitamin B complex and some vitamin C but I advised increasing that to 2 g per day. Vitamin E was given as another antioxidant for the immune system, plus the specific homeopathic remedy that I always give for cold sores, homeopathic sodium chloride, *Natrum Muriaticum* in the 200th potency. The latter remedy is miraculous in its effectiveness for curing and preventing cold sores. I usually give it once per week for prevention purposes.

From an esoteric perspective, Heather showed a depletion of energy in the heart chakra with disturbance to the thymus gland, plus slight excess of energy in the solar plexus. I understood these disturbances to be related to the strain of her teaching job. Her lymphatic system also showed disturbed energy. The esoteric healing included the standard chakra balancing, vitality triangle, immune triangle, lymphatic drainage, and the chest triangle of force to strengthen her heart chakra (see the end of this chapter and appendix 1).

Heather returned after one month, feeling much better and with no further cold sores. She was taking her raw juices regularly each morning and coping with work without getting tired. Her remedies were repeated at monthly intervals for the whole year and she had no relapses. At one stage, she had tender breasts and slight lymphatic gland swelling, but this soon cleared. After the twelve months of treatment, she noticed an unpleasant odor before her menstrual cycle, and I added a deep-acting homeopathic remedy to the liver and lymph drops; the problem disappeared. From my viewpoint this phenomenon was part of her retracing back through the inherited miasms or predispositions that her iris picture had indicated. This means that the gonorrheal miasm surfaced and this affected her menstruation; the odor was corrected when an antigonorrheal remedy was administered.

This is an ongoing case, but soon I will be able to reduce her medication. She should stay on the antioxidants for immune strength and take the herbs whenever there is any glandular swelling. Heather's is a good case to illustrate the interrelated factors in a resistant infection: work factors that affect the heart and solar plexus chakras; inherited factors affecting the immunity; and the toxins (as seen in the iris) that probably related to poor diet and poor elimination in her earlier years.

Glandular Fever

Glandular fever (mononucleosis) is another condition that occurs when an individual is stressed and lacking in immunity. The most common age for this condition appears when adolescents are in their last years of study at high school. I have treated dozens of young people with glandular fever in this age range. It can be a slow moving condition without natural treatment, and a person can continue unwell for months with recurrences for years; it can severely handicap the young sufferer in their studies and social life.

Although glandular fever is not considered to be infectious, there is an associated virus known as cytomegalus, which will usually be demonstrated in sufferers via a blood test. Symptoms include headaches, sore throats, swollen glands, and extreme tiredness. With prompt treatment using natural therapies, the clients are usually on their feet and much improved within two weeks, even after a severe attack.

Glandular Fever Case Study: Shelley, 12, came to my clinic after having symptoms of glandular fever for two weeks. Her glands were very swollen, and initially she had needed cortisone for an extreme allergic reaction to the virus, such that her throat was too swollen even for her to drink. This was an unusually severe reaction. The previous year, she had suffered a bout of pneumonia, so it is likely that her resistance was low from that period on.

Her iris was moderately fine in structure and only indicated slight lymphatic congestion; her diet was moderately good, so it appeared that stress was the main factor, although she was not yet in her last years of school. As with many immune disorders, I found, when doing the energy scan, that the energy in the thymus gland was disturbed, plus there was deficient energy in the heart chakra, which conditions the thymus gland.

The esoteric healing included the chakra balancing and vitality triangle, the immune triangle to help the thymus gland, the chest triangle of force to tone the whole chest area, the lymphatic drainage technique, and the opening triangles, which involve the throat chakra and arms.

Her prescription included vitamin C (2 g daily), homeopathic liver and lymphatic cleansing and toning drops, the colloidal minerals iron phosphate and potassium chloride for the glands, and a mineral tablet for energy, combining magnesium, calcium, and potassium phosphate with high doses of vitamin B complex. In addition, Shelly had a mixture for her lymphatic glands, containing equal parts of burdock, cat's claw, catmint, violet leaves, and dandelion (to act as a bitter tonic for her digestion).

When Shelly returned in one month her mother reported that she had started to improve within two days following the first visit. The esoteric healing was repeated, plus she was given the same prescription and homeopathic drops for her sinus. She had two more visits at monthly intervals, and remained good in all respects. The treatment period was four months. One year after Shelley's first visit, her mother brought her older son, 15, with the same problem. She reported that Shelley was in good health.

A case of glandular fever like Shelley's, in her teenage and final years of school, is a typical example of the effect of stress on the immune system. I treat more cases of glandular fever at this age than for any other age group. The continual demands of study seem to affect the thymus gland, and this made Shelley succumb to the virus, not infectious in the usual sense. Again, we can see the relation between the inner factors of stress and possible deficiencies, such as vitamin C and particular minerals. If Shelly had had sufficient vitamin C and a strong and clean lymphatic system, she would most probably have been resistant to glandular fever. It was especially noteworthy that, in connection with the heart chakra, which governs the lungs, she had previously suffered pneumonia, involving the lungs.

If an individual does not have adequate treatment for glandular fever, I have found that they often suffer from congestion of their lymphatic glands and various respiratory problems for years afterwards. From a naturopathic viewpoint, glandular fever only occurs when immunity is weak, and, unless it is strengthened with a holistic approach the individual is prone to suffer repeated viral attacks. They often have recurrence of the symptoms they suffered during the glandular fever, such as swollen glands, sore throats, headaches, and tiredness.

Second Case Study: Suzy, 36, was such a case. She had suffered glandular fever at 17, and visited me while suffering a constant cough. She was very tired and experienced flu-type symptoms whenever she had dietary indiscretions, although her diet was usually very good. She had a history of thrush (Candida infection) and her menstrual cycle was elongated. Her iris revealed moderately heavy lymphatic congestion; when I did the energy scan of her organs, I found a disturbed energy field in both the lymphatic system and the thymus gland, plus insufficient energy flowing through the heart chakra. Esoteric healing for Suzy included the chakra balancing, vitality triangle, immune triangle to correct the energy in the thymus, and the lymphatic drainage technique. This sequence was repeated at each visit.

Her first prescription included an herbal mixture with catmint, red clover, centaury, cat's claw, and astragalus; homeopathic drops; colloidal minerals iron phosphate and potassium chloride for cleansing the lymph glands and toning immunity; and magnesium and potassium phosphate in colloidal form for improving her energy levels. She was already taking vitamin C, and she increased this to 2 g daily.

Suzy did not notice much difference during the first month. She traveled interstate at this time and had a poor diet. At her return visit, her energy field was still disturbed in respect to the lymphatic glands and the thymus. She had suffered thrush the whole month, and her hair was falling out. Her prescription was repeated, and I prescribed her acidophilus capsules for the thrush and homeopathic drops for her thyroid, which I found to be out of balance (thus causing hair loss).

This was the turning point. She had no further viruses or thrush, her hair stopped falling out, and her menstrual cycle became regular. Recently, she said her health remained good.

Suzy returned for another visit recently, and was delighted to tell me she was twelve weeks pregnant. As often happens with the change in hormone levels during pregnancy, she had a relapse of thrush. She also wanted treatment for an accumulation of mucus. I gave her an herbal mixture, consisting of olive, clivers, and burdock for the thrush;

the antioxidants vitamin C and E for protection during pregnancy; colloidal calcium phosphate for the bones of her baby; and liver and lymphatic drops for lymphatic cleansing combined with homeopathic Ipecachuana drops, which are given for the nausea of pregnancy.

Chronic Fatigue Syndrome

Chronic Fatigue Syndrome (CFS) has perhaps become a clinical sign within humanity of the level of pollution in our environment. Many persons are incorrectly diagnosed by natural therapists, or sometimes by self-diagnosis, as having CFS. Many people think that if you are continually tired and not responding to natural therapies quickly, then you must have CFS. It is a difficult condition to diagnose, because there is no accepted differential diagnosis to distinguish CFS from other somewhat similar syndromes. It does very often appear to follow glandular fever.

From my viewpoint, CFS is a sign that one's immunity is severely compromised. CFS is due to an accumulation of toxins in the connective tissue (muscles, ligaments, and joints). These toxins are what some clinicians call a "wild protein." This protein molecule is considered to be a mixture of viral particles, antibiotic material that has not been correctly metabolized by the liver, and, perhaps, antibodies to this foreign material. These molecules clutter up the connective tissue, causing inflammation, pain, and weakness. I first came across this theory in a booklet on toxicology from a German homeopathic company called Reckeweg. I wondered if this theory coincided with the small brown toxic spots I was starting to see within the iris of the eyes of many individuals from the 1980s onwards.

I have found it interesting to study the iris of such individuals. Very often, there are many dark-looking toxins, spreading out from the area in the iris corresponding to the digestive system and into the areas corresponding to the connective tissue. In particular, there are tiny dark brown dots superimposed on the general brown areas. These tiny brown dots are significant. I often see such dots in people who do not have CFS, but who have symptoms of toxic overload in certain areas of the body, such as the digestive organs or joints.

The main defining symptom for CFS is pain in many muscles, especially on exertion, and severe impairment and exhaustion from walking and from any physical exertion. Many people come to my clinic with exhaustion, but this is often nervous exhaustion. Individuals suffering CFS have a more deep-seated exhaustion than that, one that penetrates all cells, due to the toxic overload.

The ideal way of removing these toxins is to improve a person's vitality to the stage where they can throw a fever to burn up the waste. This is a long process, and, very often, CFS clients have done the rounds of dozens of therapists and medical people before they get to me. They often suffer severe depression. This is understandable, whether it is from despair and frustration at there being no cure or from the actual effect of toxins on the brain. I nearly always find that the energy of their thymus gland is impaired.

CFS Case Study: Alise, nine, was my first case of chronic fatigue syndrome, presented to me at a time when the term had not even been coined. I described her case then as post viral muscle problems, with a degree of dystrophy in the muscles of her limbs. She was first brought to me in early 1987 by her mother, who had received naturopathic treatment at my clinic. I am pleased to use this case, because as CFS can run such a long course, it is useful to report on a case that has remained well for many years.

Alise began her illness with bronchitis, and despite some naturopathic treatment, it progressed to pneumonia. After receiving antibiotics, she still did not regain her health after the lungs cleared, and began to have muscle pains and weakness. When she was brought to see me, she could hardly walk and tottered into the consulting room at a very slow pace. At the time, I had not started to use esoteric healing, although I was doing scanning. I was doing an energy evaluation using the Vega instrument. This is an electronic diagnostic machine that measures the biological age of the person and their organ function.

In the case of Alise, her biological age was about 48, despite her chronological age of nine. For her first prescription Alise was given homeopathic drops to antidote the flu virus that led to her pneumonia; drops to tone her liver so that it would detoxify the toxins in her system; a zinc salt for her immune system; vitamin C and colloidal minerals iron phosphate and potassium chloride that her mother had given her throughout the illness; vitamin E for muscle strength; a blood cleansing herbal tablet containing red clover, burdock, and poke root to clean out the muscle toxins; vitamin B complex and colloidal potassium phosphate for energy; and an herbal rheumatic tablet.

Despite this array of supplements, Alise only made very slow improvements over the first five months of treatment, although her biological age (via Vega testing) was now 36 years—still high for a nine-year-old. The turning point seemed to be when I gave her homeopathic drops to antidote previous immunizations. I used the energy scan and discovered that her legs were completely lacking in normal energy flow. I then carried out certain techniques (see *The Vivaxis Connection*, Hampton Roads, 2000)[50] and noted the return of energy through her legs. These techniques used energy flows from the Earth to restore bodily energies. After these two measures, Alise made slow, but steady, progress.

For some years, she stayed on these basic remedies, although I added colloidal calcium phosphate for strengthening her muscles. Her biological age became normal, and she only suffered muscle aching after a lot of exercise or walking. As a teenager she stayed on a maintenance dose of colloidal calcium, magnesium and potassium phosphate, vitamin E, liver and lymphatic draining drops, and vitamin B complex. After she left school, Alise did veterinary science, with a view to combining this approach with natural remedies and, on completion of her course, she married. She still needs to have a maintenance course of remedies from time to time, but has remained well.

Most of my CFS clients are not prepared to persevere for this length of time. This illustrates the problems with modern living, and how toxins are gradually accumulating in the connective tissue of some individuals. Such persons are probably predisposed to CFS, to some extent, by the health of their parents and by inherited factors. My clinical viewpoint is that we have multiple factors leading to CFS: heredity, poor immunity associated with previous illnesses, such as glandular fever, pneumonia, and multiple childhood immunizations, plus nutritional and environmental factors.

Autoimmune Diseases

So far, we have discussed simple immune situations, for which the basic approach is improving diet and giving a boost to the immune system. Esoteric healing is usually added to this, especially in the case of adults. However, an increasing number of diseases are being classed as autoimmune disorders, and these include rheumatoid arthritis, lupus, ulcerative colitis, multiple sclerosis, Hashimoto's disease, scleroderma, and Human Immune Deficiency Syndrome, commonly known as HIV. In these diseases, the body's immune system destroys its own tissues. Obviously, these are not simple immune situations.

There is as yet no clear understanding as to why this self-destruction occurs. In some instances, such as in rheumatoid arthritis, lupus, and Hashimoto's, there is a familial incidence of the problem, but only certain family members are affected. From a naturopathic viewpoint, those who suffer autoimmune disease may have a triggering factor, such as poor nutrition, severe stress, or a virus. From an orthodox medical viewpoint, it is thought that destructive antibodies are formed after the immune system goes on defense alert following a viral attack.

In autoimmune diseases, the antibodies start to attack the body's own tissues, such as in Hashimoto's disease, where antibodies attack the thyroid gland, or in multiple sclerosis, where the myelin sheath covering nerves is destroyed. In the case of lupus, the destruction can be very widespread in the body and may affect joints, kidneys, heart, and brain.

From an esoteric viewpoint, autoimmune disease is intimately related to the health of the heart chakra and its related gland, the thymus. In most cases of autoimmune disease, I find an energy disturbance in this gland that often returns whenever the client is under stress. My theory is that, in time, it will be discovered that the thymus gland controls the whole immune system and is related to both cell mediated and humoral immunity.

From an esoteric viewpoint, autoimmune disease is intimately related to the health of the heart chakra and its related gland, the thymus. In most cases of autoimmune disease, I find an energy disturbance in this gland that often returns whenever the client is under stress. My theory is that, in time, it will be discovered that the thymus gland controls the whole immune system and is related to both cell mediated and humoral immunity. Hence, any deep grief or disturbance in the heart chakra may be the initial cause as to why the immune system becomes unbalanced, with antibodies attacking cells and tissues or killer cells going out of balance with suppressor cells.

It is only fairly recently that the pineal gland was found to be the conductor of the endocrine "orchestra," so who knows what is yet to be discovered about the equally mysterious thymus gland. The next case illustrates some of my clinical experience with the thymus gland and immunity, in the area of lupus.

Lupus Case Study: Teresa, 56, came to me for healing, but did not initially want naturopathic treatment. A melanoma on her leg was removed in 1993, followed by infection of the leg. She has suffered from lupus since she was a young woman in her midtwenties, and her kidneys, heart, and joints were affected by the disease at various times in her life. When she saw me, she had severe impairment of the right hip and an ulcer on the surface of her right foot, giving her considerable pain. She had undertaken a lot of healing work on herself over the years, and had a very positive attitude to her problem. Throughout her health ordeal, she has worked as a drama coach.

On scanning her energy field, I found that all the chakras were exhausted and undersized, and that the chakras of the right hip and foot were completely blocked. Her thymus, liver, and lymphatic system were all disturbed. The healing work I did included the immune triangles, lymphatic drainage, and work on removing old thought-forms that were associated with the root chakra. Thoughtforms (crystallized, stagnant thoughts and attitudes) can be attached to any chakra and result from persistent thoughts, amounting, sometimes, to an obsession with some problem from the past.

The owner is not always aware of having these old thoughts. I use a visualization technique to draw the thoughtform away from the chakra and destroy it. It would not be wise for a new practitioner of healing to undertake this technique without the supervision of a well-trained teacher, because these thoughtforms can attach themselves to the healer if not properly destroyed.

After four healings at weekly intervals, Teresa's chakras had returned to a more normal size, and the hip and foot chakras were open. Teresa was sleeping better, and the thymus gland and lymphatic system were improved. During the healings, she often had significant insights about why she suffered from lupus and what she needed to do, in a psychological sense. She was a delightful client to work on, because she was so sensitive to energies.

I persuaded her to take an herbal mixture for her foot ulcer and her immune system. She had resisted taking any herbs because of fear that some herbs would overstimulate the immune system. In fact, echinacea, in her case, would have caused a problem. I carefully matched the herbs to her energy field, using a dowsing technique, and she checked my selection at home herself, using a similar technique with a pendulum. The mixture consisted of red clover, catmint, cat's claw, clivers, and motherwort, all in equal parts.

After two months on this mixture, Teresa's ulcer had healed. I then persuaded her to take an herbal anti-inflammatory tablet for her hip, and this greatly improved the pain in her hip. She also started taking magnesium orotate (400 mg) for the pain and spasm in her body, and a general antioxidant that included vitamins A, E, and C. She was able to give up taking analgesics (painkillers) for her hip and began to walk without a stick. It is possible that she will eventually have to have the planned hip replacement, but she is now in a much better state for surgery. Teresa has taken a new job as a speech therapist and feels she will find the strength to cope with its challenges.

It is a joy to be able to improve the general condition of some of these very chronic ailments even though we know that autoimmune diseases are, to some extent, incurable. If we can replace orthodox drugs with simple medicines that have no side effects, and if we can restore the person to health sufficient to have a satisfying life, then we have achieved an important contribution to their well-being.

The Chronic Miasms and Autoimmune Disease

In the area of autoimmune disease, it is most likely that the afflicted person has certain inherited tendencies called chronic miasms. What homeopaths call the syphilitic miasm is the inherited tendency most closely related to autoimmune disease, for it is related to destruction of tissue, and this is a prominent feature of such disorders. The syphilitic miasm means that a forbear in one's childbearing years, perhaps several generations earlier in the family tree, suffered syphilis. Even though the infection is not inherited by subsequent generations, there will be predispositions towards destructive processes in the body that are related, according to homeopathic theory, to the original conditions of that illness.

Whether we consider multiple sclerosis, rheumatoid arthritis, Hashimoto's disease of thyroid, or lupus, there is destruction of tissue by the body's own antibodies. It is likely, therefore, that all persons suffering autoimmune disorders have a basis of this miasm in their family tree that may go back many generations. Some current triggering factor, such as nervous stress, grief, a viral attack, poor diet, or environmental stress, sets the conditions of the disease, but it's based on the old predisposition.

Every now and again, one has a client presenting with what seems like such a formidable collection of health disorders that even my optimism in the value of natural therapies, combined with subtle healing, somewhat dwindles. Sally was such a case. It is bad enough to have a serious autoimmune disorder like lupus without having it combined with two other life-threatening conditions. Sally is still in the relatively early stages of natural treatment for several chronic disease processes, but her improvement has already been so outstanding that it is worthwhile describing her situation to date.

Second Lupus Case Study: Sally, 38, arrived at my clinic with her husband in July 2000. Sally and her husband conduct food demonstrations for healthy living; she is also a trained singer, longing to be well enough to continue with that occupation. She had lupus, a life-threatening reduction in blood platelets (thrombocytopenia), deep vein thrombosis, osteoporosis, and severe migraines with each period. She also has uterine fibroids. Due to taking large doses of cortisone to help restore her platelet levels, she had gained 42 pounds in six months; this treatment also predisposed her to calcium loss and osteoporosis.

So here we had a very contradictory situation. Sally's lack of platelets caused her to be in danger of hemorrhage and she had a drug for this condition. On the other hand, she had a tendency to clot, for which she needed to be on the anticoagulant Warfarin, which needs to be monitored, in case she bled to death. With this dichotomy of problems, you can imagine I hardly knew where to start.

As in the previous cases, when doing the energy scan, I found a disturbance in the energy underlying the thymus gland. In addition, she had disturbances throughout the digestive tract and also underlying the pituitary, thyroid, adrenal glands, ovaries, and uterus. There were corresponding chakra imbalances, involving the heart, throat, and sacral areas. The esoteric healing each month included chakra balancing; vitality triangles for energy; blood circulation work for the thrombosis; lymphatic drainage stimulation for general toxins; the immune triangle for the lupus; the sacral triangle for her menstrual pain; and the opening triangles for her throat to help her singing voice. I took particular care to be gentle with the circulation technique because she had the history of thrombosis, and it is possible to be too forceful and cause a clot to move around.

I noticed that as the months went by, Sally's chakras became more even, in terms of their energy flow, and that restored them to a normal size. When she first came for treatment, they were undersized due to a lack of energy flow probably over a long time. Remember that the energy spins through a chakra, and this determines its size when measured from side to side. Each healing gave Sally's chakras a boost, so that in combination with the natural remedies she took over time, they maintained a normal size.

For her first month's treatment, I gave Sally an immune and lymphatic toning mixture, containing the herbs astragalus, catmint, cat's claw, red clover, and burdock, and the tissue salt *Kali Muriaticum* for removing excess fibrinogen in the blood, in this case, directed towards the clot in her leg. Vitamin E is another essential ingredient for dissolving the clot, and I gradually increased the dosage of this from month to month. The capacity for vitamin E to dissolve and prevent the formation of clots was established as early as the 1930s. I gave Sally liver and lymphatic toning drops for detoxification, including Thuja in homeopathic form to resolve the inherited tendency to form fibroids. For her energy and severe migraines, I gave her the nerve-balancing combination of the tissue salts potassium phosphate and magnesium phosphate, together with vitamin B complex.

It was interesting that Sally had suffered a lot of grief over criticism and estrangement from her family. From my perspective this had caused a disturbance to the heart chakra and, thus, to the thymus and immune system. Even the clot in her circulation could, in an esoteric sense, be considered directly related to the heart chakra, for the circulation of the blood has a connection with our love nature as it is expressed through its conditioning chakra, the heart. Fortunately, Sally has a very supportive husband, and this fact helped ameliorate the danger.

On her first return visit, Sally reported much improvement. Her migraines had lessened in intensity and she had lost some weight. Her rheumatologist was very pleased with her progress. She had also improved her diet. After two months of treatment, she suffered a heavy cold, which, in my experience, is often the body's way of throwing off toxins through mucus discharge. Often in a chronic disease, the body stops having acute manifestations like colds, because it does not have enough vitality to have a cold. In the third month, Sally had no migraines for the first time in years.

When I checked her chakras during the fourth month of treatment, I found there was still an imbalance with the base chakra, which was outsized in comparison with the sacral center, and that the solar plexus was undersized. As discussed in chapter 4, in health, the chakras should be balanced and equal in size, although the overall size varies from person to person, according to their level of emotional, mental, and spiritual development. If any chakra is larger than the others there will be an excess of energy flowing to the associated organs. There can also be a feedback into the chakra from the physical side, such as after the administration of a drug that affects the glands.

So the cortisone Sally was taking was probably responsible for the enlargement of the base chakra, and her sacral may have been undersized, in relation to the congestion of her ovaries and uterus. She was still having occasional migraines (even though she had gone an entire month without one) but they were less severe and of shorter duration. Her Warfarin dosage was reduced a bit, because it was causing bleeding from the kidney.

I kept her naturopathic treatment much the same, but added an extract from wild yam to apply topically in order to restore balance between her estrogen and progesterone levels. In time, this would further reduce her weight. As discussed earlier, the estrogen of most women over thirty starts to gain dominance over the progesterone, causing many hormonal problems, including weight gain.

Sally is yet another case in which holistic treatment and a synthesis of remedies is essential. From the inner point of view, she had a destructive process that may have been started by low self-esteem, resulting from family interactions; these affected the heart chakra and its associated gland, the thymus. This may have, in turn, triggered off the autoimmune disease, lupus, which usually comes from an inherited predisposition. The administration of cortisone for lupus further unbalanced her glands (especially the adrenals and ovaries) and caused her to gain a lot of weight. The immune problems from the thymus gland disturbance may have also triggered off the platelet deficiency. Her clotting tendency perhaps related to a lack of vitamins E and C, and was, therefore, more to do with her lifestyle over a long period.

So her case was complicated, and it was necessary to treat all aspects. My clinical aim is to get her off Warfarin and cortisone and to improve her immune system, so that her lupus does not affect the vital organs. Meanwhile, after seven months of treatment, her clot was gone, according to ultrasound, and her blood tests for lupus antibodies revealed an improvement in that condition.

Both Sally and her husband are delighted at her increased energy, weight loss, reduction in migraines, and improvement in joint pain. She will need to be on natural treatment for several more years to gain optimum improvement, but considering her prognosis before this treatment had been very grim, this is not much of a burden.

I have treated enough cases of autoimmune disease by now to state that it appears there is a close connection between this problem and the thymus gland. In each case, I have found energy disturbances underlying the thymus gland, either before treatment or at some time during the course of the treatment. In many of these cases I have found the heart chakra also to be disturbed. Perhaps we will soon discover that a malfunction of the thymus hormones causes autoimmune disease, whereby the body produces antibodies that attack its own tissues.

I am certain the healthy functioning of the heart chakra keeps our immunity in balance. This must be the reason why many persons can have destructive antibodies from perhaps an inherited source, yet do not get autoimmune disorders. When the energies of the solar plexus chakra are raised to the heart through meditation and service, we gain a psychic and physical immunity that can even overcome inherited predispositions.

Effects of Electromagnetic Fields on the Thymus Gland

However, not only inherited weakness, poor lifestyle, or level of consciousness affect the thymus. We are now dealing with an unprecedented rise in background electromagnetic radiation from many sources, such as television transmitters and aerials, satellites, mobile phone towers, computer terminals, and many household and workplace technologies. Many of my autoimmune-diseased clients relapse, and I find that their thymus is disturbed when they travel long distances by airplane and receive a dose of cosmic radiation. A thymus disturbance can also happen when one is exposed to a simple gadget in the home, something generally thought to be harmless, such as a water bed, computer terminal, or digital clock close to the bed,[51] as the next case shows.

Thymus Disturbance Case Study: Rosalind is a delightful 74-year-old woman who has been consulting me for thirteen years. She attributes her general good health to the naturopathic treatment I have given her over these years. She originally saw me in 1989 for an autoimmune disease called *Lichen planus* (inflammatory skin lesions), which is like lupus.

Rosalind had suffered sore, raised plaques on the mucous membranes in her mouth and had joint problems. She had an excellent diet and exercised regularly, so her lifestyle was good. The conventional medical treatment given to her was cortisone, which is usual for many autoimmune problems. Her earlier history included Bell's palsy, at age 30, and a duodenal ulcer when she was 44. I noted that she had a lot of mercury amalgam fillings in her mouth; this meant that her mercury levels may have been high and have contributed to her *Lichen planus*.

Her first prescription included vitamin C (1 g twice daily) and an herbal tablet featuring red clover, burdock, and poke root for detoxification of her lymphatic system and to assist immunity; vitamin A to strengthen the epithelial tissue in her mouth; vitamin B_3 to help sore gums and tongue; liver and lymphatic cleansing homeopathic drops; zinc for immunity; and homeopathic mercury to eliminate the mercury in her system. On Rosalind's return visit, the sore plaques in her mouth were much better and she continued the same prescription for a period of fifteen months, after which she discontinued treatment.

She returned at the beginning of 1995 with sore joints, a condition that had been diagnosed as Polymyalgia rheumatica. This condition is related to her autoimmune problem. On this occasion, she was given an anti-inflammatory herbal tablet; an herbal tablet with immune stimulating herbs; the colloidal minerals iron phosphate and potassium chloride for the inflammation and any fibrous processes in the joints; the colloidal minerals potassium and magnesium phosphate to balance the nervous system and, indirectly, to influence immunity; herbal drops to balance the ovaries; and the usual homeopathic drops for liver and lymphatic toning.

By this time (mid-1990s), I was adding the subtle healing to the treatment of most of my clients, and whenever Rosalind had a flare-up, I found the energies of her lymphatic and immune system (including the thymus gland) to be disturbed. Rosalind was able to gradually reduce her cortisone until she was off it completely, and, over the next few years, she came every two or three months for review and assessment. Over this period, she had a few brief flare-ups with either sore joints or mouth, but, generally, she stayed very well.

During 1998 and 1999, she had some relapses of her condition and bladder infections. The latter were greatly helped by using grapefruit seed extract, which is a powerful antibacterial agent. She also developed a slight cataract that remained under control for some time by taking homeopathic drops of silica and calcium fluoride in the thirtieth potency. By this time, I was using some new powerful immune-stimulating herbs, such as astragalus, cat's claw, catmint, and an African rheumatic herb called Devil's claw. Each time Rosalind came off her cortisone, I gave her vitamin B_5 to support her adrenal glands. I added vitamin E to her regimen at this stage, for joint mobility and as a general antioxidant.

Rosalind was going along very well when, in early 2001, she had one of her joint pain relapses. We had experienced the longest period of hot weather recorded in Melbourne, but the weather had then suddenly turned cold and Rosalind relapsed. We might take the view that this is why the joints had relapsed. However, while doing the esoteric healing, I found, as usual, that her thymus was disturbed; the thought came to me to ask whether she had started to use an electric blanket at the time her joints became painful. On questioning her later, she said that, indeed, was the case. I explained how the electromagnetic field from this electric blanket, therefore, caused the thymus gland energy to be disturbed so that the immune system became imbalanced, which, in turn, caused the inflammatory process in the joints to start again. Rosalind agreed to try bed socks and a hot water bottle instead of the blanket.

Since then, despite very cold weather (for Australia), Rosalind's joints have given her no pain. Perhaps it was coincidence, but there is no doubt in my mind that man-made electromagnetic fields can affect the thymus gland. As Rosalind gets older, her thymus gland may be more vulnerable and easily upset; this is related to her inherited tendency to *Lichen planus* and joint problems.

For some time, she has been on a maintenance supply of herbal anti-inflammatory tablets, vitamins C and E, nerve energizing and balancing minerals, and the homeopathic drops for liver and lymphatic toning. She will probably need to stay on a moderate array of supplements for the rest of her life, but she regards this as good insurance and prefers this to continual cortisone.

Stress, Immunity, and Breast Cancer

In many cases, a person comes to me after surgery and chemotherapy with the idea of preventing further tumor growth by improving their general health and immunity. Breast cancer is still a major killer of women in Western countries. From a naturopathic viewpoint, it has multiple causes including poor diet, stress, use of underarm deodorants that suppress the elimination of toxins from the lymphatic glands, accumulation of waste in the lymphatic system, and a disturbance in the thymus gland. I frequently observe a lesion in the heart area of the iris in women who have manifested breast cancer, and I often wonder if this is associated with a deep, unresolved grief.

Another concern is an imbalance of hormones, as some breast cancers are estrogen-dependent. Many women of all ages have an imbalance in the ratio between their estrogen and progesterone. This kind of imbalance was discussed in detail in the chapter on hormone disturbances, but, for here, I'll say that this imbalance underscores my concern with balancing the chakras as part of a treatment, because the glands are directly conditioned by the chakras. Thus, profound grief or stress can depress the function of the thymus gland and, thereby, affect immunity.

Breast Cancer Case Study: Joy, 42, came for treatment following a radical right mastectomy, followed by radiation and chemotherapy. She had suffered very heavy periods since, and had premenstrual tension. Sinus congestion was another problem, and she had very heavy lymphatic congestion. This was illustrated in her iris, and was also evident when I did the energy scan. Joy's diet was quite good, so I did not make adjustments in that area.

Her first prescription included an herbal tablet, with cat's claw and echinacea, vitamin C, and a homeopathic liver and lymphatic remedy for the immune system, and high-potency vitamin B complex, with colloidal magnesium and potassium phosphate for energy. She was also given wild yam extract, as a topical cream, to balance the hormones. After the usual chakra balancing and vitality triangles, I did the techniques for the immune system (triangle of thymus and adrenal glands), plus the lymphatic drainage techniques to help clear the lymph.

After one month on this treatment, Joy had a bit more energy and the treatment was continued. She had esoteric healing each month, which concentrated on the lymphatic and immune systems. After the second month of treatment, Joy reported that her periods had shortened in length and their pain had lessened, but she had a sore back, so the Bowen treatment was included for this problem. Her use of supplements continued.

Joy had a heavy cold after an international trip, but her periods continued to improve. Her back needed Bowen treatment from time to time, over the next few months. She continued treatment for two years and, during this time, went back to study for an arts degree to complement her teaching work. She had a lot of strain (a parent diagnosed with cancer) but managed to complete her studies. She had another bad viral infection, and I switched her herbal tablet to a mixture, with red clover, dandelion, clivers, burdock, and catmint to give the immune system an extra boost. It is expected that a person who has had long-standing lymphatic congestion will continue to suffer a virus from time to time.

Joy went back to primary teaching after her studies were partially completed. This occasionally caused some back problems, due to lifting her small students. She has remained generally well, and her specialist is pleased with her progress. This case shows how natural therapies can be a good health insurance following a serious health challenge and during a subsequent period of considerable stress.

When discussing possible psychosomatic causes of her cancer, Joy said that she realized, following her tumor development, that she had far too little rest and relaxation in her life. She reflected on how she rushed continually in this direction and that to ferry her children around, apart from her work stresses. She now has a different attitude towards life, and incorporates relaxation on a regular basis.

Summary: In summary of heart chakra conditions, we remember the connection between the heart chakra, thymus gland and physical heart and circulation. As with the other glands, the thymus can be conditioned by the heart chakra, and can also be affected by environmental factors, such as electromagnetic fields. The thymus gland is intimately related to our immunity and the maturation of white blood cells that fight aberrant cells, such as cancer cells, bacteria, and viruses in the body. Other physical factors affecting the thymus gland and heart include inherited predispositions and, of course, our general lifestyle, with respect to diet and exercise.

We have looked at cases that include the physical heart and circulation, as in blood pressure, and have then considered cases involving the immune system, from simple infections to serious autoimmune processes. Some of these cases have highlighted the possible effect of the emotions on the heart chakra, with subsequent flow on in the physical body.

Healing Practice for the Heart Chakra and Chest Area

There are a number of exercises we can do for the heart. The circulatory exercise is best learned under an instructor, because it needs to be learned very carefully, so as not to use too much force. The exercises that we will cover here are the blood pressure triangle, a triangle for the immune system, and the chest triangle of force, which I use for all heart, breast, and chest disorders. It strengthens the chest area and allows energy to flow freely through the whole area. It is also very useful to bring in love energy for a grieving person.

1. Align as previously described. Place your hands on the client's shoulders and imagine linking up with your own soul, the client's soul, and the source of all healing and ask that healing take place according to the plan of the soul.

2. Visualize the healer's flow of energy by imagining the following alignment—soul, heart, head, and hands.

3. When you sense that the energies are flowing, move to the left-hand side of the client and kneel or sit so that you can comfortably have your hands on either side of their body. From this point on, you do not physically need to touch the client.

4. Balance all the chakras up the spine, as described earlier, by placing the right hand behind the spine of the client and the left hand in front. Sense the impact of the energies on the hands and move them gently in and out, in an accordion fashion, until the flow of energies seems balanced between your two hands.

5. Balance the chakras, in the order of solar plexus, base, sacral, heart, and throat. During this process, there is no need to have the hands close to the body. It is best to have them as far away as possible, because it seems to be easier to assess the energies in this way and is less disturbing to the client.

6. Now move a few feet in front of the client and do the **immune triangle** as follows. Connect your brow chakra, in imagination, to the client's thymus gland, situated just above the heart and the hand chakras, one to each adrenal gland, situated just above the kidneys.

7. Connect the three points with light and wait until the energy flows. This exercise stimulates and balances the thymus gland and adrenal glands in a way that also balances and stimulates the immune system (see figure 20).

8. Next, do the **chest triangle of force,** which is useful for strengthening all structures within the chest cavity, including the heart and thymus gland. Use the hand chakras to balance between the throat center and the throat minor center just below it. This is a straight line, rather than a triangle. Hold these two points until you sense a balance between them.

9. Connect your brow chakra with the heart chakra of the client, then connect the hand chakras with the breast minors and connect these three points with light, waiting, as usual, until the energy is flowing.

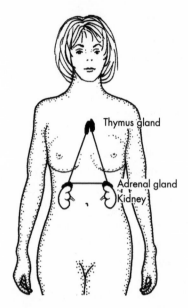

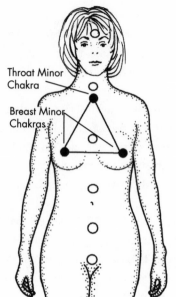

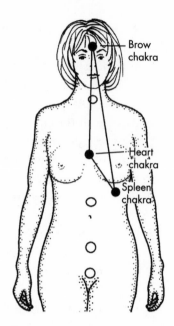

FIGURE 20: THE IMMUNE TRIANGLE. The immune triangle is used for promoting immunity, especially in cases of autoimmune disease. A triangle is visualized by the healer between the thymus gland and adrenal glands of the client.

FIGURE 21: THE CHEST TRIANGLE OF FORCE. The chest triangle of force connects the throat minor center and the breast minors. Before visualizing this triangle, an initial triangle is made between the breast minors and the heart center.

FIGURE 22: THE BLOOD PRESSURE TRIANGLE. The blood pressure triangle connects the brow chakra, heart chakra, and spleen chakra.

10. Vitalize the actual triangle of force by keeping your brow chakra with the client's throat chakra, and use the hand chakras to connect, in imagination, one with each breast minor. (The breast minors are just above the nipples, as in figure 21.)

11. Connect the three points—throat minor and breast minors—in light and wait for the energy to flow (see figure 21).

12. To vitalize the **blood pressure triangle,** connect the following points in the client: brow chakra, heart chakra, and spleen chakra. Connect, in imagination, your brow chakra with that of the client, and use one hand chakra to connect, in imagination, with the heart chakra of the client and the other to connect with the spleen chakra.

13. Visualize these points to be connected by light, and wait, as usual, until the energies are flowing between the three points (see figure 22).

14. Close as in the previous exercises.

11 *The Throat Chakra and Lymphatic Conditions*

The next chakra to consider is the throat chakra and its associated disturbances. The related endocrine gland is the thyroid, and the relevant tissues are the larynx, upper lungs, bronchial tree, and the lymphatic vessels and glands. Consequent disorders that we will explore in this chapter include thyroid problems, and all those illnesses that involve a congested lymphatic system. These include eczema, tonsillitis, asthma, bronchitis, and more serious conditions, such as the spread of cancer into the lymph glands.

The throat chakra is intimately associated with our creative expression, and when this is blocked or not used in an appropriate way, thyroid problems can occur. However, there can also be a strong inherited predisposition to thyroid problems; this tendency can be triggered off by frustrated creativity or other psychological states that can affect the thyroid. From a nutritional point of view, a person may have an underactive thyroid from lack of iodine in the diet. So you can see how holistic we need to be in treating this area of the body, to include subjective factors, inherited tendencies, and lifestyle including nutrition.

In relation to the connection between the throat chakra and the lymphatic system, I often find throat chakra congestion when there is a lymphatic problem, such as eczema or bronchitis. We need to study the lymphatic system so as to understand the various disorders resulting from its disturbance.

The lymphatic system is a network of vessels and glands, distributed throughout the body tissues. In particular places, such as the armpits, groins, neck, breasts, and abdomen, there are collections of small lymphatic glands that, in health, are hardly perceptible to palpation. Most people will remember how, during an infection, they had an enlarged gland somewhere, which, to touch, felt like a pea or almond-sized lump. This is the reaction of the lymphatic and immune system to the infection, and the swelling is caused by a congestion of white cells that the immune system sends to fight the infection, plus a degree of inflammation. Due to its surveillance function, the lymphatic system is often known as the "policeman" of the body.

In naturopathic philosophy, the tonsils (situated in the throat) are known as the gateway to the lymphatic system. If this collection of lymphatic tissue called the tonsils is healthy, ingested virus and bacteria are often stopped from progressing further into the body by the action of the white blood cells resident in the tonsils. Other similar lymphatic structures are the adenoids, situated at the back of the nose. This tissue can deal with bacteria and viruses we breathe in.

Many people have their tonsils and adenoids removed in early childhood, following repeated infections of the tonsils. However, these organs should be left in place, if possible, as they are the first line of defense against inhaled bacteria and viruses. Many individuals commence a cold or influenza infection with a sore throat, and this alerts us to the possible physical connection between the throat, throat chakra, and the lymphatic system. Note that often people come down with an infection when they have used the throat a lot in lecturing and teaching, activities that deplete the throat chakra of energy. Conversely, if the throat chakra is well energized, it has a positive conditioning effect on the whole lymphatic system.

Flowing in the lymphatic channels and through the lymphatic glands is a clear fluid called lymph. This contains various nutriments derived from the digestion and also, when necessary, white blood cells, with antibodies on their surface to deal with infection. The lymph bathes the various tissues and drains them of toxins, which are taken away to be metabolized by the liver. Unlike the circulation, there is no heart to pump the lymph around through the lymphatic channels, so it is dependent on body movement. This means that we need adequate exercise for a healthy lymphatic system, otherwise, the lymph stagnates and the lymphatic glands can start to become congested.

From a naturopathic view, if we have swollen lymphatic glands, it is a sign that the body needs to undergo a cleansing process, as otherwise, stubborn infections are likely to develop when we contact bacteria or viruses. Hence, a natural therapist takes the opposite view from most orthodox practitioners, who would see the glands becoming congested only after contact with infection or, in the most serious situation, from infiltration by cancer cells.

The spleen, an organ the size of your closed fist, is found below the left ribs and is indirectly related to the lymphatic system. It acts as a storage for blood, produces antibodies, and is also a destroyer of worn-out blood cells. In conditions where there is a great excess of white blood cells, as in malignancies like lymphomas and leukemias, the spleen becomes very congested.

From a naturopathic view, if we have swollen lymphatic glands, it is a sign that the body needs to undergo a cleansing process, as otherwise, stubborn infections are likely to develop when we contact bacteria or viruses. Hence, a natural therapist takes the opposite view from most orthodox practitioners.

In this chapter, we start with skin problems, like eczema, associated with a congested lymphatic system, and then move to more chronic lymphatic problems, such as bronchitis and cancer, before discussing some cases involving the endocrine gland associated with the throat chakra, the thyroid.

Acute Skin Inflammations

A healthy body eliminates waste daily through the bowels, kidneys, skin, and lungs. When the metabolism is sluggish and/or the lifestyle, including nutrition, is poor, toxins gradually accumulate in the lymphatic system. If the vitality is high, the body will often endeavor to eliminate waste through the skin. In other words, the body's inherent vitality appears to have a centrifugal action, as far as the toxins are concerned; the toxins come to the surface via the thousands of small lymph channels under the skin and are "spun" out of the body. This is the first stage of disease, according to naturopathic principles, as was described in chapter 6.

The level of vitality in a person with eczema can usually be gauged by the iris, such that, when vitality is high, the iris fibers will be fine, straight, and close together. Eczema cases often exhibit small white or yellowish dots and clouds around the periphery of the iris, and this illustrates congestion in the lymphatic system. These marks gradually disappear as the problem clears. You will often see a dark ring around the edge of the iris, which indicates a sluggish skin action. This means that the skin rarely sweats and is, therefore, unable to eliminate waste coming from the small lymph channels under the skin via the sweat. This waste then gradually accumulates in these small lymph channels. If the body has good vitality, the skin can become inflamed as a means for eliminating the underlying waste, according to naturopathic philosophy.

Unfortunately, it is socially unacceptable to have a rash on the skin, so the sufferer rushes for medical assistance, and cortisone cream is often used to suppress the inflammation. This has the effect of driving the toxins deeper into the system, and is one reason why eczema is often followed by, or alternates with, asthma.

The alternation between eczema and asthma is really a switch between the first and second stage of disease, according to the diminishing level of vitality in the person. So when vitality is high, the lymphatic system carries the toxins to the periphery (the skin) and eczema can be the result. When the person is tired, or develops a respiratory virus, or perhaps has an immunization, immunity is compromised, the energies lowered, and lymphatic toxins sink deeper, and are often eliminated as mucus from the nose, throat, vagina, or lungs, as in asthma.

The philosophy of the medical profession is that both eczema and asthma are examples of Type 1 sensitivities to foreign protein, but the natural therapist is looking at deeper causes related to the lymphatic system.

Eczema

Cortisone and other suppressive treatments rarely cure eczema. Cleansing the lymphatic system with herbs, plus supporting the immune and nervous systems with minerals and other natural supplements, can permanently resolve eczema. There is often an inherited predisposition to eczema, but this can be resolved with deep-acting homeopathic remedies.

It is interesting that I rarely find subjective problems with eczema in children, so the need for esoteric healing does not feature so strongly in this condition. Often, the lymphatic system will temporarily register a disturbance, and sometimes the liver is disturbed and congested. Logic suggests that when an ailment is on the surface of the body, unless there are other accompanying deep-seated disturbances, there will not be deep-seated energy problems coming from the psyche. So, with eczema in children, I do not usually find the need to do the esoteric healing, providing I use constitutional homeopathic remedies to deal with the inherited tendency for the skin problem. I frequently use esoteric healing with adult eczema cases, as there are usually other accompanying ailments related to chakra disturbances. Eczema and asthma frequently run in families and thus illustrate the miasmatic tendency, as discussed in chapter 3.

I have observed that eczema, recurrent colds, and asthma in young children appear to be triggered, in many cases, by immunizations. This is always a controversial subject, and if parents give their babies and small children extra vitamin C (up to one gram daily, depending on their age) for at least a week before and for several weeks after immunization, any negative effects may usually be minimized. Immunization is given to produce antibodies against particular infectious diseases that the child may encounter in its environment. This is, therefore, an appropriate place to briefly mention a few further facts about the immune system.

Eczema Case Study: Adrian, three, had suffered eczema since birth, and it worsened by age five months. This could have been related to the usual compulsory immunizations that start when an infant is six weeks of age in Australia. I have often noticed that eczema worsens after immunization. When treating babies, I always ask about their milestones, as this gives valuable information for selecting the right homeopathic remedy. Milestones were out of the usual sequence in this case—Adrian teethed and crawled before the usual age but he walked later than average. This gave me a clue to the type of his inherited predisposition (Adrian's father also suffered eczema), so I selected barium iodide in a high potency as his constitutional homeopathic remedy.

I also gave Adrian sulfur, in a moderately high potency, every second day for the itch of eczema; homeopathic liver and lymphatic cleansing drops; colloidal calcium (which I find is essential for childhood eczema); and a chewable vitamin C tablet. His diet was not too bad, but I advised his mother to keep him off wheat, as many people with skin problems cannot digest wheat properly; sourdough rye bread is a good substitute. He was already on soymilk, instead of dairy products. I suggested he take a teaspoon of flaxseed oil twice daily to help with his skin. This oil helps the skin in many ways, chiefly because it is rich in omega-3s, which help dry skin and reduce inflammation of the skin.

Over the next month, Adrian made a lot of improvement, and the bad patches in the flexures of his arms and legs started to diminish. Incidentally, eczema in these positions is a sure sign of the need for colloidal calcium. Adrian was unusually compliant at taking his remedies and, after the second month, I decided to give him an herbal mixture, because he had one bad asthma attack during his second month of treatment. This mixture was based on clivers, red clover, burdock, catmint, and cat's claw. I also changed his deep-acting homeopathic remedy to calcium iodide. At his next visit, his mother reported that his skin had continued to improve and, after six months, we started to taper off the treatment.

Both this and the next case were resolved fairly speedily, compared to many of the other ailments described in this book. This is because, as mentioned, people with eczema have fairly good vitality and, therefore, the treatment can be comparatively speedy. This is more obvious with children, yet it can also apply to adults.

Second Case Study: Sam visited my clinic with a rash of six months' duration. She had taken cortisone orally for five days, but with no improvement. Her father had skin problems while she had a history of asthma and hay fever. This is pertinent, as it illustrates the retracing phenomenon discussed in chapter 3. Her body had successfully managed to undertake two stages of this retracing process, but appeared to be stuck at the final stage. Sam mentioned that her skin rarely perspired, which was a clue to why the toxins under the skin were being retained.

Her iris indicated an inherited weakness in the bronchial area on the left side, lymphatic congestion, and the need for balancing the nervous system. Sam is a teacher, so she has a challenging job and, thus, a stress input. Her diet was fairly balanced vegetarian fare, and my main suggestion was to cut out bottled orange juice, because it has an acid effect on the body, as distinct from freshly squeezed orange juice.

Her first prescription included an herbal cleansing mixture, with catmint, clivers, dandelion, red clover, and motherwort; colloidal minerals magnesium and potassium phosphate for the nervous system; and sodium and calcium phosphate for an acid tendency and for the weakness of tissue involved with the bronchial area, as observed in the iris. The usual cleansing homeopathic drops for liver and lymphatic toning were prescribed. She was already taking vitamin B complex.

Sam enjoyed the esoteric healing, which was directed towards cleansing the lymphatic system and balancing the endocrine system, as she was postmenopausal. Each healing, therefore, consisted of balancing the chakras, the vitality triangles, lymphatic cleansing and the endocrine pentagon—pituitary, adrenal glands, and ovaries (see appendix 1). During the healing, Sam always saw a lovely shade of purple/blue and felt heat in her hands. Some people feel heat in those parts of the body that have been disturbed by their ailments. I often think that when people have heat in the hands, it is a sign that they could be good healers. Sam's rash cleared up completely during the first month of treatment, although we still worked on improving her mineral status for another six months.

It would be wonderful if all cases resolved as easily as this one. Despite the fact that there was an inherited disposition and a history of deep-seated lymphatic problems, as in her previous bronchitis, Sam's eczema was resolved very quickly. This was, in part, due to the current good lifestyle of Sam, in terms of her diet and general wellbeing.

Earlier, I discussed the progression of disease from the acute stage, through sub-acute, to chronic. We could class a yearly cold with inflamed sinuses and throat as an example of an acute infection, whereby the body uses a passing virus, in conjunction with its immune system, to create inflammation and produce mucus discharge. When I was young and had very dramatic eliminations of mucus associated with colds, I noted that I always felt better *after* the cold than before. I remember thinking, perhaps we forget how well we feel before a cold. But, in fact, after such an elimination of mucus, we feel *better* because the body has eliminated a lot of waste and concurrently increased its vitality. We will now consider common respiratory problems, including acute and sub-acute manifestations, as these are situations in which the vitality is lessened to some extent.

Respiratory Problems

If we consider the most common health problems that interrupt our life, both at work and play, it would have to be those created by upper respiratory viruses, such as colds and flu. The average person has at least one cold per year, and children in their early years, especially, usually have a number of colds and viral infections per year. The medical profession tells us that it is "normal" for children to suffer a number of viruses when they first become exposed to many other children at kindergarten and elementary school. However, the severity of such infections varies enormously, and many children succumb to asthma attacks following a virus. As mentioned in the previous chapter, one-in-four Australian children are asthmatics and carry their "puffer" (inhaler) to school each day. This prevalence has given Australia the title "asthma capital of the world."

While most colds and influenzas are not life-threatening, they cause a high absenteeism at school and work, and can be very inconvenient for weddings, examinations, concerts, and socializing. It is necessary for the immune system to have regular challenges but, from a naturopathic viewpoint, the unpleasant response to such challenges can be minimized by holistic treatment.

Other respiratory problems involve more recurrent ailments, such as the chronic bronchitis that develops from constant uncontrolled chest infections in heavy smokers. There are various causes of the chronic obstructive pulmonary disease that develops in life-long smokers and miners, or for the rare conditions such as asbestosis, for those who have been exposed to asbestos in various industries. Lung cancer is one of the major causes of death in most countries and must, therefore, also be included in this section.

We will start our journey through respiratory system problems with the tonsils, as they are the gateway to the lymphatic system. It is normal for the tonsils to be large in young children, because these glands are the gatekeepers for the deeper parts of the lymphatic system. The medical profession now accepts that the tonsils have a role to play in immunity, and they do not automatically remove them as before at the first sign of swelling. If the tonsils become infected, it indicates that the lymphatic system is congested; after the lymphatic system is cleansed with herbs and homeopathic remedies, the tendency to tonsillitis disappears.

Naturopaths have found that certain substances must be present in reasonable quantities within our tissues to prevent or cure infection. At the top of the list is vitamin C, and individuals use up this vitamin in variable amounts, according to the physical stress of their external and internal environments. For instance, if you live or work near an area with lots of petrochemical fumes, you will need more vitamin C than someone living and working in the countryside. This is because vitamin C is used up in your body to oxidize poisons and toxins from chemicals, drugs, or bacteria.

Recent research has indicated that vitamin C is able to positively affect the white cells in the blood that are associated with immunity.[52] Nobel prize-winner Irwin Stone established decades ago that vitamin C is associated with electron transfer in the cell. In other words, it is intimately associated with energy in the body, and natural therapists are dedicated to improving vitality so that the body may be more resistant to disease. I often say that if I were allowed to use only one substance in my practice, it would probably be vitamin C. Although our body uses up this vitamin in varying amounts, a sensible dose for an adult on a day-to-day basis is one gram in the morning and another at night. During infection, this may need to be increased to 10 g or more per day, or to bowel tolerance level, which means until bowel actions become loose.

Another main consideration for immunity is the state of the liver. This is the organ that has to metabolize all the toxins taken into the body, even such substances as the contraceptive pill or hormones in hormone replacement therapy. You can imagine that in the twenty-first century of polluted cities and unnatural diets, our livers are under great biochemical strain. In my clinic, I routinely prescribe liver detoxification for every client, in the form of a homeopathic mixture of three liver herbs: St. Mary's thistle *(Carduus Mar)*, greater celandine *(Chelidonium)*, and fringe tree *(Chionanthus)*, all in a low potency of 6x.

I usually mix these liver homeopathics with eight other homeopathic remedies for cleansing the lymphatic system. The lymphatic homeopathics include the remedies *Sarsparilla*, *Juglans Reg.*, *Hepar Sulphuricum*, and *Fumaria*, all in low potencies. The client receives a one-ounce bottle, containing the liver and lymphatic homeopathics and takes seven drops twice daily, sometimes over many months, to detoxify. These are the liver and lymphatic toning drops mentioned elsewhere in the case studies in this book. These liver and lymphatic herbs are also often used in a 1:2 liquid extract, but the homeopathic mixture is suitable for very young children who will not take strong-tasting herbs.

In addition to vitamin C and the liver and lymphatic drops, I use herbs such as clivers, burdock, red clover, catmint, and cat's claw when the immune system's vitality is very low. I usually give the herbs in equal parts as a liquid mixture, in doses of 5 ml, twice daily. Sometimes, in place of a mixture, I give the client capsules of echinacea in doses of 3 g, taken several times daily. If you are traveling or unable to bear the taste of herbs, this is a more suitable form. Research has shown the efficacy of echinacea in helping to resolve respiratory infections; however, the lesser known, but equally easily available, herb burdock was reported as early as 1958 to resolve staphylococcal infections effectively, even in low dilutions.[53]

Another frequently needed supplement for immune vitality and resistance to infection is zinc. Due to farming methods and poor diet, a number of people are deficient in zinc. An Australian company has produced an interesting way to tell whether a person is deficient in zinc: it's called the Zinc Tally test. The client is given 10 mls of the zinc solution to hold in their mouth; if no flavor is experienced after 10 seconds, they need zinc. Those who do not need zinc experience a strong unpleasant metallic taste almost immediately. Several manufacturers of natural therapies have produced products combining vitamin C, echinacea, and zinc, to be used to combat infection.

Tonsillitis Case Study: Darren, 18, suffered repeated sore throats with infected tonsils, usually on the left side, and the condition seemed to be greatly aggravated by eating anything containing yeast and white flour. He had a history of asthma. His diet was only fair, but he was making an attempt to eat more whole foods and to eliminate yeasty items like pizza. His iris indicated a great accumulation of toxins in the gastrointestinal tract and connective tissue. Such toxins, as defined by iris diagnosis, appear in a hazel-colored eye as darker brown discolorations and spots.

If we are free of toxins, the iris should be the same clear color from its edge in to the edge of the pupil. This is rarely found today, but when I was first in practice in the early 1970s, I often observed older persons who had been born early in the twentieth century to have good constitutions along these lines. Unfortunately, the bodily accumulation of toxins by people born in the second half of the twentieth century has been considerable.

Toxins, as illustrated in Darren's iris, were surprising, as his mother is health conscious and was adamant earlier that his diet as a young person had always been good. So it seemed a mystery as to where these toxins were originating. However, I was also treating Darren's father, who showed similar iris patterns, and it seems likely there can be an inherited *tendency* to accumulate toxins. Darren's allergies may also be related to this inherited predisposition.

From the esoteric perspective, my etheric scan indicated energy disturbance in the lymphatic system and congested energy in the throat chakra. Darren also discussed the fact that he felt his study caused stress that, at times, affected his throat. You will remember that stress from study can be a prelude to glandular fever cases. Esoteric healing included the chakra balancing, lymphatic cleansing, especially in the throat area, and nervous system balancing, featuring the vagus triangle. (The lymphatic triangle used in the esoteric healing is described at the end of this chapter.)

My naturopathic treatment for Darren included vitamin C at 2 g daily, to be increased if he suffered tonsillitis; magnesium orotate, 400 mg, twice daily, for spasm in the gut from the allergies; liver and lymphatic toning homeopathic drops; an herbal mixture containing meadowsweet and marshmallow for toning and soothing the digestion; and red clover, sarsaparilla, and clivers for the immune system and lymphatic cleansing.

I also gave him flower essences, for negative emotional states: Mimulus for fear, Hornbeam for strength of mind and body, Larch for confidence, and Rescue Remedy as a general tonic. The flower remedies were mixed together in a small bottle, to be taken as five drops, three times daily. I have found that the flower essences work directly on the chakra system, and, presumably, this is why they can resolve various emotional states.

On his return visit in a month, Darren reported an improvement in digestion and said he had had only minor sore throats. During the third month, he had a flare-up of tonsillitis, and he always had a bit of a relapse during this treatment period if he ate yeast or white flour products. This meant he had to be very strict with his diet as many biscuits, cakes, and baked products contain refined wheat flour.

At this stage of the treatment, I also gave him particular homeopathic phenolic remedies to resolve his problem with wheat and yeast. There are phenolic substances in many plants in our environment, and they often are concentrated in our foods. Some people are allergic to these molecules if exposed to large concentrations of them in a food or in the environment. Most foods contain phenolic compounds of one kind or another, and some people develop hypersensitivities to such compounds in foods or plants.

All together, Darren's treatment took twelve months, but the intensity of it tapered off as he improved. The interesting features in Darren's case include the relationship between study stress, his digestive processes in connection with allergic reactions to particular foods, and the effect of poor digestion on his lymphatic system. Accumulation of waste in the lymphatic system is a common result from poor digestion. The disturbance from stress affected his throat chakra, which added to the disturbance of the lymphatic system from the subjective side. The prescribed treatment, therefore, addressed the inner and outer factors.

I have observed in my clinical practice that the majority of individuals who suffer repeated and severe respiratory infections have poor nutrition. In particular, their diet often lacks vitamin C, and often emphasizes many refined foods. White flour and sugar products may predominate over vegetables, fruits, and whole grain cereals and breads. We call this a mucus-forming diet, meaning that the body gradually accumulates toxins that manifest as an excess of mucus. When such an individual suffers a cold, instead of it running a brief course, there is often a long period characterized by infected mucus with discharge from the nose and coughing and mucus discharge from the bronchial tracts. In children predisposed to asthma, this is a further possible complication. I also treat many adults with asthma, and the following case is one in which the symptoms cleared up quickly with natural therapies.

Asthma Case Study: Jane, 25, developed asthma after moving to Melbourne at the age of 12. She was always worse in winter, and took a bronchodilator medication as necessary, especially before exercising. She suffered a rash on the face and had recently contracted chicken-pox. Her energy was poor, and she often had severe premenstrual tension with mood swings, despite taking the contraceptive pill. Her diet was fairly good, with whole grain cereal for breakfast, soymilk, a salad sandwich for lunch, pasta, lentils, tofu, and a small amount of meat for dinner. Her iris had a moderately open structure and her autonomic nervous system, as illustrated in the iris, had been obviously under stress for many years. This could have been due to a mineral deficiency as illustrated by the open structure of the iris. Typical of many of my clients, her iris revealed she had a lot of acid in her body.

Jane was already taking vitamin B complex and vitamin C. Her first prescription from me was an herbal mixture, containing cat-mint, cat's claw, and red clover for clearing her lymphatic system and boosting immunity; dandelion for her liver toning; hops and oatseed for energy. In addition, I gave her the homeopathic liver and lymph cleansing drops and colloidal calcium, potassium, and magnesium phosphate to restore her mineral status. I also gave her esoteric healing, with an emphasis on lymphatic drainage and the chest triangles, after the chakra balancing.

At her return visit in a month, she reported her glands were still swollen and that she had suffered a bad cold with some asthma. However, she had more energy, and this had enabled her to go back to studying. We always prepare clients to expect that they may feel worse before they get better, and a heavy cold in the first month of treatment is very common. The important fact here is that Jane reported having more energy. This is a sign that her body could throw off the toxins. At her third visit, Jane reported much more energy, no PMS, and no viruses or asthma. Her esoteric and naturopathic treatments were continued for six months. She has subsequently remained well, with good energy, only mild colds from time to time, and little need for her asthma medication.

This is yet another case that indicates the complexity of a congested lymphatic system, exhaustion, and, in Jane's case, menstrual problems, which can also result from a lymphatic system problem. Although her diet is now balanced, I suspect it was far from balanced in childhood, as suggested by the loose pattern of the radial fibers in her iris. This weak iris structure often indicates poor mineral status. Her rapid progress with treatment suggested that subjective factors were minimal.

With asthma, after about six months, the treatment is usually tapered off, unless the person is under extreme stress through work or family problems. We advise all individuals who have a history of recurrent viruses to take 1 g of vitamin C twice daily and to increase this up to about 6 g daily, and to take up to 3 g of echinacea three times daily at the first sign of infection.

In the long term, an improved diet can make a difference in our vulnerability to infections. In the short term, I find that a course of vitamin C (1 g, twice daily), echinacea capsules (3 g, twice daily), and the tissue salts iron phosphate and potassium chloride in colloidal form can cut short the length of a cold during the stages of inflammation and elimination of mucus. Herbs such as licorice, white horehound, marshmallow, and wild cherry bark can be used for coughing. This regimen will usually minimize any secondary infections of the ears, sinuses, or chest so that antibiotics are very rarely needed. Over a period of six months or so, clients are often given a course of vitamin C, the tissue salts just mentioned, and an herbal mixture of four or five herbs to strengthen their immune system and clean out their lymphatics.

Recurrent Colds Case Study: Of all the childhood complaints I see at my clinic, the most common are recurrent colds and coughs. In many cases, there is an extension from these to asthma or infected ears. Nicholas visited me with a history of eight upper respiratory infections per year since the age of four, for all of which he was prescribed antibiotics. He produced large amounts of mucus with each infection and had previously suffered two bouts of pneumonia. His diet was fair, and his iris revealed moderate lymphatic and digestive toxins. This was a case I considered did not need esoteric healing. However, I combined the naturopathic treatment with the Bowen technique for the benefit of energy balancing via the meridian system, as it works on trigger points that balance the body via the muscles.

The naturopathic medicines I gave Nicholas on his first visit were 300 mg of vitamin C twice daily for immunity; a multivitamin and mineral tablet twice daily to gradually correct a number of possible mineral deficiencies; colloidal iron phosphate and potassium chloride for the first two stages of inflammation; an herbal mixture for immunity containing cat's claw, red clover, burdock, dandelion, and white horehound for immunity; and homeopathic liver and lymphatic toning drops.

During his first month of treatment, Nicholas had a virus, but managed without the antibiotics usually prescribed, in case he suffered a secondary infection. His mother was very happy about this. During the second month, he had another mild virus, but no cough; the third month was similar. I had explained to mother and son that he would probably continue to have some viruses until the treatment had resolved the mucus in his body, but the rewarding fact was that Nicholas no longer spent weeks away from school being sick, and today he feels well.

I have included this case because it is a good example that shows how a severe lymphatic problem can sometimes be resolved with well-chosen oral medications plus Bowen Therapy. You may wonder why no esoteric healing was needed; in a sense, it was given, via the Bowen technique. This technique works on various acupuncture points that have a reflex action on the chakras. So, although I did not specifically work on the chakras, the end effect of both the naturopathic treatment and Bowen Therapy was to work holistically on Nicholas.

We cannot discount the effect of weather on the incidence of respiratory infections. Although some individuals suffer a cold or influenza in summer, the majority succumb during the cold months. Over the last winter, I had a number of clients, including the following case, who made appointments after suffering a hacking cough for more than a month, despite several rounds of antibiotics.

Chronic Bronchitis Case Study: Shane, 40, complained of a cough, which always came with a cold every winter for twenty years. He was worse in cold air, and discharged green and yellow mucus. His diet was poor: he went without breakfast and ate no fruit, hardly any vegetables, but lots of white bread, meat, potatoes, and pasta. His iris indicated a good constitution, except for a build up of acidity in the tissues, so I was able to conclude that his poor nutrition was a major factor in his reduced immunity. He was coughing every couple of seconds during the first consultation, such that I wondered if he was headed for pneumonia.

His first prescription included vitamin C (twice daily); the tissue salts iron phosphate and potassium phosphate (five times daily); echinacea capsules (3 g, three times daily) for immunity; and magnesium orotate (400 mg, twice daily) for bronchial spasm. I gave him an herbal mixture including red clover, white horehound, licorice, wild cherry bark, marshmallow, and drosera (5 ml, four times daily).

Like most of my clients, Shane received esoteric healing. I nearly always find when I do the etheric scan on individuals with respiratory infections, that the energies in the lymphatic glands under the arms and frequently down the side of the neck are disturbed. When I mention "disturbed energies," I refer to energies that are chaotic, rather than the normal "pulsation" that I find underlying healthy tissues. Shane's esoteric healing, therefore, included the usual chakra balancing, vitality triangles, the lymphatic drainage to the bronchial area, and the immune triangle.

After two weeks, he was hardly coughing and was making an effort to eat more vegetables. He had also removed dairy food from his diet. His treatment was continued for another two months, and he did not relapse during this time. However, his future immunity will depend on whether he can improve his diet.

I am often amazed at how quickly older people suffering long-standing complaints will respond to natural therapies. This indicates that throughout life, the body can revitalize itself when given the right foods.

This case is one in which the long-term outcome will depend almost entirely on Shane having a better diet and lifestyle. His iris indicated a good constitution, and this means that he did not have inherited predispositions towards bronchial problems. Nor did his work involve much mental strain, as is very often the case in both adolescent and adult bronchial problems.

I am often amazed at how quickly older people suffering long-standing complaints will respond to natural therapies. This indicates that throughout life, the body can revitalize itself when given the right foods, as the next case illustrates.

Second Bronchitis Case Study: Don, 72, was a client for a few months, for treatment of bronchitis, in the early 1990s. When he initially visited me at age 64, he had a history of pneumonia, and this had left a degree of bronchiectasis, which is a permanent dilation of the bronchus such that a tendency to infection occurs in the bronchial area. After the pneumonia, he was given large doses of cortisone and antibiotics before coming for naturopathic treatment. This produced improvement over two months.

Don returned for further treatment some years later, after a build-up of infected mucus. Don's iris revealed deep-seated lymphatic congestion as the basis for the mucus, while my energy scan indicated disturbance underlying the liver and right lung. I gave Don 2 g of vitamin C daily for immunity; liver and lymphatic toning drops for cleansing those tissues; colloidal iron phosphate and potassium chloride for inflammation and mucus respectively; and an herbal mixture containing licorice, red clover, marshmallow leaves, euphorbia, and white horehound as a chest tonic and lymphatic cleanser.

The esoteric healing included the usual chakra balancing plus lymphatic drainage, the use of the immune triangle, and the various chest triangles (described at the end of this chapter). When Don first visited me for treatment (in 1993), I would have hesitated to suggest such healing to a businessman, but since then I have found that response is good from almost everyone despite a diversity of backgrounds. The last ten years have introduced the general public increasingly to the advantage of keeping an open mind about the validity of subjective events.

After one month, Don was feeling better and the mucus had almost disappeared. The prescription was repeated twice, and Don's improvement was maintained.

Don was a delightful person for me to treat because, unfortunately, it is unusual for an older person to have such an optimistic and positive attitude. His diet was good, and after his presenting problem of phlegm was resolved he preferred to stay on minimal treatment and to visit me to preserve the improvement. I think this is a good idea because, at age 72, his bronchial weakness from his earlier pneumonia will tend to attract new infections. So, although the elastic lung tissue may not be restored, he need not suffer further infection.

Persons with chronic bronchial problems, such as in emphysema and bronchiectasis, in which elasticity of lung tissue or bronchial tubes has been lost, need to take supplements over a long period of time. But if they are suffering from continual infections, as in the case of bronchiectasis, this is usually worthwhile. Some individuals who have suffered bouts of pneumonia will also succumb to this respiratory weakness. It is often long-term smoking that causes emphysema, that is, loss of elastic tissue in the lungs.

Another type of chronic respiratory problem with mucus, but less life-threatening than the others, is sinusitis. Many people get infected sinuses on a regular basis or, if it is not infected, they have a chronically blocked nose. Often there is an allergy to milk products, so one of the first suggestions I make to anyone who suffers from sinus problems is to replace dairy with soy products.

Sinusitis Case Study: Ravi visited me in 1997 for a number of problems, including chronic digestive upsets featuring discomfort and gas. As a young child, brought up in Asia, he had suffered from malaria and diphtheria. He had a very demanding career and traveled a lot, to educate seamen on avoiding human errors in their work. His sleep was poor, and he had suffered chronic catarrh of the nose with yellow mucus discharge all his life. His ears were also blocked, and this would not have been helped with the constant flying. It is interesting that he had the digestive problems, because I often find that an accumulation of mucus begins with poor metabolism of foodstuffs, even in people with a good diet. Ravi's diet was fair, but emphasized cheese.

At his first visit, I gave him vitamin C (1 g, twice daily), liver and lymph homeopathic toning drops, and a capsule for the sinus, containing horseradish, garlic and echinacea. In addition, I gave him a zinc compound (zinc also helps with immunity) and homeopathic drop for his enlarged prostate gland, and the tissue salts potassium and magnesium phosphate for his nerves and sleep problems.

His energy field was disturbed in the area of the sinuses, the lymphatic glands in the neck, liver, and prostate gland. Ravi received the usual chakra balancing and lymph cleansing technique, plus specific triangles to improve his energy level. On his next visit, he said his nose was clear for the first time in decades, and it has never relapsed. Due to his incessant travel, his digestion was a problem from time to time, especially after he had a mild attack of hepatitis A. Over the next few months I gave him an herbal digestive mixture containing meadowsweet, gentian, cranesbill, and dandelion; these are bitter and tonic herbs for the digestion.

Ravi kept on the treatment and visited me every two months for a check up for nearly three years. He regarded the treatment as health insurance to fortify his hectic life. From time to time, I changed the treatment.

He no longer needed the stomach mixture after a few months, and then I added the tissue salt sodium phosphate for heartburn and he took that as needed. I continued him on the basic treatment for his sinusitis of vitamin C, sinus herbs, and drops throughout this period.

In summary of Ravi's case, I would say that his childhood medical history of malaria and diphtheria predisposed him to catarrhal problems, including the blocked sinus and ears. As he had an Asian background, his diet as a child may have been very poor. His stressful career, with constant travel and lecturing, affected his throat chakra and lymphatic system further, and the poor diet while traveling disturbed his digestive system. Prostate problems are common with men over 50. His treatment needed to be holistic to cover all these factors. The naturopathic treatment attended to his early poor health and current lymphatic problems, and the esoteric healing helped the stress.

I have noted that when a person is able to keep in regular alignment with their soul via some skill such as meditation, they manifest a type of magnetic radiance that keeps their immune and lymphatic systems in good working order via the conditioning chakras.

You can see from the variation of symptoms between these cases of lymphatic congestion that there is a certain complexity involving the relationship of the ailments described to other chakras, as well as the throat. There is sometimes an inherited factor; there are lifestyle factors, such as diet and smoking; and then there are emotional and mental factors that condition the lymphatic system via the chakras. As mentioned, the throat chakra conditions the lymphatic system; however, if the lymphatic system is congested from addiction to junk food or nicotine, then the solar plexus (desires) and the sacral center (appetites) will also be involved. In the case of severe infection related to the lymphatic system, the heart chakra, via the thymus gland, will also be involved.

We come now to cancer, which is the most serious disorder that can involve the lymphatic system, and all the above-mentioned factors can be involved.

Cancer

The following case of cancer had dietary, environmental, and lifestyle factors that conditioned a poisoning of the lymphatic system. This case is one of the most spectacular treatment outcomes I have encountered in my thirty years of naturopathic practice. Regardless of whether the original and preliminary diagnosis of cancer was correct or not, the patient was severely affected in his respiratory function at the time of his first appointment with me.

Lung Cancer Case Study: Frank, 60, came to my clinic at the end of March 1999. He had been a smoker for 46 years, and had developed a continuous cough. The previous week, he had been drowsy and suffered fever and shaking. On taking his history, I learned that Frank was a printer by trade and had been exposed to benzene over many years in the form of solvents. Other aspects of his lifestyle with a negative impact on his health included taking 40-45 spoons of white sugar daily, dispersed through 10-15 cups of tea. His diet was poor in other respects, with white bread and cornflakes as his only cereals. His smoking and constant craving for sugar indicated addictive traits in his personality, but he was a cheerful person and did not seem to have any particular worries now or in the past. His wife did most of the worrying. He had just given up smoking following his diagnosis of advanced lung cancer.

Frank's iris diagnosis was interesting, as it showed a lack of minerals and tone, particularly in the lung and bronchial areas of his body, plus a large accumulation of acid waste throughout all his tissues. The autonomic nervous signs indicated in the iris showed considerable imbalance, which meant that, despite his happy-go-lucky disposition, there was much stress in his nervous system. This was related, in part, to his environmental pollution from chemical solvents and cigarettes.

A blood test revealed moderate anemia and a raised blood sedimentation rate, which usually indicates chronic disease of some kind. The more specific diagnosis of computerized tomography (CT scan) revealed a 1.7 inch x 2.5 inch cancer mass of the right lower lobe of the lung and a mass measuring 1.2 inch in the left upper lobe. The report concluded that "the findings are most consistent with right lower lobe primary bronchogenic carcinoma and possibly left lung metastasis." A biopsy was suggested prior to having surgery or chemotherapy. Frank's doctor suggested to his wife that his prognosis was very poor, and he received no conventional medical treatment.

I prescribed the following natural remedies for Frank the day after the first CT scan: antioxidants vitamins C and E, betacarotene, and the colloidal minerals iron phosphate, potassium chloride, potassium phosphate, and magnesium phosphate. These minerals were given, respectively, for anemia, fibrous (or scar) tissue resolution, and to enhance vitality. Frank took an herbal tablet twice daily to improve his immune function; this included cat's claw, echinacea, astragalus, and goldenseal. I included bovine tracheal cartilage to prevent aberrant cell division and to improve immune function.

I instructed Frank to drink fresh carrot, apple, celery, and beet juice at least twice daily, to eat wholemeal bread instead of white, and to cut down his sugar intake as soon as possible. Although he was coughing continually, we managed to conduct a session of esoteric healing at his first visit. His energy field showed considerable disturbance of the immune and lymphatic systems, with local disturbances in both lungs; his liver energy was also disturbed. After the chakra balancing, I worked with the immune triangle (lymphatic system, respiratory system, and liver). The throat chakra, throat minor chakra, and lung triangle all featured in each healing (see end of this chapter).

At the next appointment three weeks later, Frank had nearly stopped coughing, and he had curtailed his sugar intake. He was feeling—and he looked—much better. On inspecting his energy field via my usual scan, the disturbances previously noted had resolved. His wife telephoned excitedly two days later, after his first biopsy, and read out the report. The findings were that he had degeneration of the cells lining the lungs and a possible blockage of part of the respiratory tree, but there was no mention of malignancy. After this biopsy, Frank was given a course of antibiotics.

Frank continued to flourish, and a further CT scan resulted in the medical comment that "the two regions of abnormalities within the lungs are once again seen but have continued to decrease in size suggesting inflammatory aetiology." From a naturopathic view, inflammation is the opposite pole of malignancy, and if there had been some kind of resolution of a tumor, we would expect an inflammatory stage. A further X ray in a few months indicated that his lungs were completely normal, and his blood tests for hemoglobin and sedimentation rate had also become normal within two months of naturopathic treatment.

After six months of treatment, I stopped the herbs and the bovine tracheal cartilage, but continued vitamins C and E to help prevent free radical damage to his lung cells in the future. I added a preparation of hydrogen and oxygen, in drop form, to eliminate the acidity in his system. After another few months, I streamlined his treatment to a maintenance dose of vitamins C (2 g daily) and E (300 IU daily), and a mineral salts tablet, combined with vitamin B complex.

Frank continues the maintenance treatment and looks and feels exceedingly well. It has been a struggle for him to keep off the sweets. He traded his syrupy tea for many sweets per day during the third month of treatment. Further discussions about the possible biochemical results from such a high sugar intake reaffirmed his commitment to healthy eating. The mineral chromium was given once per day to help with sugar craving, and Bach flower essences were added to balance his emotional states, in respect to cravings. After he had been well for two years, I noticed his acidity levels creeping up, according to iris diagnosis, and I found he was now addicted to having two chocolate-coated ice creams every day. I suggested flavored and frozen yogurt, in moderate amounts, as an alternative.

During the last two years, Frank had a general checkup with me every two months. During the first two years of treatment, he suffered severe respiratory infections from time to time, which was expected from a naturopathic viewpoint. There would have been a lot of toxic material in his body and, as his vitality increased, this would be eliminated via mucus during and following an infection. During these phases, he was instructed to have large doses (6–10 g daily) of vitamin C, initial 2 hourly doses of his tissue salts iron phosphate and potassium chloride, and 6 g of echinacea, three times daily.

This case is a good example of the retracing phenomenon whereby Frank went from cancer, the most chronic stage of ill health, back to the sub-acute stage with a lot of mucus discharge. Interestingly, he also had a fairly dramatic skin rash after two years on the treatment program. This was effectively treated by adding an herbal mixture for one month. So, in fact, we could say there was evidence of Frank retracing back through the main three stages of his disease. He has been well, thus far, for over four years.

There were no deep-seated negative emotions to deal with in this case of apparent malignancy. His lung problem seemed to be very much "weighted" in the direction of pollutants from the environment, smoking, and poor diet. From my point of view, this is one of

the main reasons why Frank made such a spectacular and uncomplicated recovery.

Cancer is a complex condition with many causes, and I consider
that, in each case, there is an inner and outer factor that varies in proportion from person to person. The previous case had no complicating factors from nervous and emotional stress,
and we could almost say that smoking and work
chemicals were the major outer factors for the
disease. The inner or subjective factors appeared
to be minimal, and perhaps that was the reason
Frank's progress was so rapid.

> *The throat chakra and its expression, via the thyroid gland, mirrors the expansion of communication systems throughout the globe, because the throat chakra rules our means of communication via the larynx or voice box. Anyone with an inherited tendency to thyroid problems will be more vulnerable in this twenty-first century of speed communications as compared to a century ago.*

Thyroid Imbalances

We will finish this chapter with two cases
related to imbalances of the thyroid gland, the
outer expression of the throat chakra. Remember
the connection between the governing chakras
of these two glands, the ovaries and thyroid? I
think the increase of thyroid problems is directly
related to the increase of energies flowing
through the thyroid as humanity becomes more
creative, in a mental sense, and energies move
from the sacral center to the throat center. This
is causing a temporary instability in the gland.

The throat chakra and its expression, via the
thyroid gland, mirrors the expansion of communication systems throughout the globe, because
the throat chakra rules our means of communication via the larynx
or voice box. Anyone with an inherited tendency to thyroid problems
will be more vulnerable in this twenty-first century of speed com-
munications as compared to a century ago.

Hyperactive Thyroid Case Study: Veronica, 34, came to me suffering from hyperthyroidism, which means she had an overactive thyroid. In such a case, the metabolism is speeded up. She had
palpitations, a fast pulse, panic attacks, insomnia, and was losing
weight. Earlier in her life, she had had an underactive thyroid, and
another family member also had thyroid problems. Her life had been

stressful, as one of her two children has the genetic disorder called Down's syndrome and is moderately retarded. Veronica's doctor had put her on the usual medication for "killing off" some of the thyroid, but she sustained unpleasant side effects from this medication and wished to have natural treatment, instead.

Veronica was an intelligent and sensitive person, and I find this often goes with throat chakra overstimulation and thyroid problems. Thus, she was not prepared to put up with the negative attitude of the first doctor she consulted and took responsibility for her own health, despite dire warnings from this particular doctor. However, she also had the tendency to worry a lot on behalf of those she felt responsible for, and this was, at times, very exhausting for her, as it can cause a tendency toward overactivity of the throat chakra.

Veronica's general lifestyle was healthy, and her iris indicated a fairly good constitution. The autonomic nervous system, which governs the endocrine glands, was disturbed, and there was a marking in the left iris that corresponded to the position of the thyroid gland. This indicated an inherited tendency to the problem. An energy scan revealed a disturbance in the throat chakra and thyroid gland. Her naturopathic treatment included magnesium orotate (400 mg, twice daily); tranquillizing herbs for the panic attacks; homeopathic kelp and magnesium iodide in the thirtieth potency for the thyroid; and liver and lymph cleansing drops for general detoxification. I also gave her flower essences for calming the emotions.

After applying the chakra balancing and vitality triangles, I focused on the thyroid gland and the opening triangles. The opening triangles are the throat center and shoulder minor centers, throat center and elbow minors, and throat center and hands. Visualizing these centers on ourselves or others brings any blocked or excess energy in the throat center out via the arms, to be expressed creatively in some way (see the end of this chapter for the practice instructions).

On her return visit in two weeks, Veronica reported that the palpitations were gone. Her pulse was back to normal, despite reducing the drug given by the medical doctor, though she was still having some panic attacks.

In another two weeks, she had undergone further blood tests, which indicated that the thyroid gland was nearly back to normal, although the thyroid-stimulating hormone from the pituitary was still slightly imbalanced. It was interesting that the throat chakra was now underactive, as compared with the other chakras, when I did the energy scan. It is common for the thyroid gland to become temporarily underactive after previously being overactive. It seems that the chakra was reflecting this change. Subsequent checks revealed that all the chakras were in balance. On her fourth visit, I worked on the head glands, including the pituitary. Her basic physical supplements were continued.

On her fifth visit, Veronica had no clinical symptoms, and I could not find anything out of order in her system. A blood test revealed that her thyroid and pituitary were both normal in terms of their secretions. This meant that the thyroid-stimulating hormone (TSH) from the pituitary gland was now at the normal level of secretion. When the thyroid is overactive, the level of TSH drops to compensate, so as to reduce stimulation of thyroxine production in the thyroid. In keeping with a return to balance, Veronica's thyroid secretion had lowered and returned to normal levels. You can see here the interplay between the pituitary gland and thyroid.

Her panic attacks were over, and she asked if it was safe to get pregnant again. I could not see any barrier to this, as there were no contraindications to pregnancy with any of her natural supplements. She became pregnant almost immediately, but suffered bad morning sickness. I gave her homeopathic drops for this, and they gradually alleviated the problem.

Two months later, Veronica was found to be carrying triplets. Perhaps the creative energy from the thyroid gland was flowing in an unexpected direction! I increased her mineral intake to accommodate this challenging situation of growing three babies. Three apparently healthy baby girls arrived when Veronica was thirty weeks pregnant, and the pediatrician was satisfied with their birth weights and health.

Veronica's case indicates the influence of the mind on the throat chakra, and the effect of mental overactivity on the thyroid in the presence of an inherited predisposition to thyroid problems. This overactivity manifested, at times, in a clear and discriminating intelligence and, at other times, in worry. She was always very sensitive to energies and during the pregnancy of the triplets had talked about their presence as "overshadowing souls." Unfortunately, one of the triplets later died as a result of a malformed heart, and this was a time of great grieving for Veronica. However, her thyroid did not relapse, in part, due to the backstop of physical remedies and the esoteric healing that was continued when necessary. So both the outer and inner factors were addressed in her case.

The doctor, who on my referral, had been monitoring Veronica, was impressed with her progress and referred another thyroid case to me. Lou's case was different because it involved not only a disturbance in the thyroid hormone, but some microzymal antibodies, which are present in autoimmune diseases of the thyroid. If these are in excess, they can attack the thyroid and eventually render the thyroid underactive when there is no healthy tissue left. This problem is called Hashimoto's disease, and the sufferer may need to take thyroid hormone replacement for the rest of their life.

Hypoactive Thyroid Case Study: Lou was 33 when she was sent to my clinic. She was fourteen weeks pregnant, and my energy scan indicated a disturbance in her thyroid gland and throat chakra. The iris indicated moderate toxins in the gastrointestinal tract, although her current diet was good. Blood tests revealed a moderate level of the destructive antibodies just described and an elevated level of thyroid-stimulating hormone (TSH), which meant that the pituitary gland was trying to stimulate the thyroid gland.

I gave Lou an herbal mixture to normalize her immune system, including red clover, clivers, cat's claw, *pau d'Arco*, and lemon balm; colloidal sodium and calcium phosphate as important mineral supplements for the growing fetus; vitamin C as a general immune balancer and detoxifying agent; vitamin B complex and a homeopathic nerve tonic for energy; and homeopathic toning drops for the liver, lymphatic glands, and thyroid. After a couple of months on this regimen, further blood tests indicated that her thyroid function had improved and her energy was also improving as a result. After another few month's of treatment, the blood tests for thyroxine levels and microzymal antibodies were completely normal. This meant that the destructive antibodies were no longer present and the secretion of thyroxine was at the normal level.

I gave Lou esoteric healing during each visit. After the chakra balancing and vitality triangles, I concentrated on the chest triangle of force (the breast chakras and throat minor), as this can strengthen the thyroid; I also used the immune triangle to resolve the problem of the destructive antibodies. The lymphatic drainage triangle was included, to cleanse the area around the throat. It is interesting to sense the response of the unborn baby to these healing procedures. During the last two months of her pregnancy, the baby moved strongly in the uterus when I thought of connecting with its soul, and there was an atmosphere of joy surrounding Lou at these times.

After the healing session, when I compared notes with Lou, it appeared that she felt the baby move strongly about the time when I thought of connecting with its soul. Like Veronica, Lou was sensitive to spiritual energies, and was conscious of her children as souls connected with her own.

As a general note, it is important to do the esoteric healing gently, especially during the early months of pregnancy, and it is not advisable for persons untrained in these methods to treat pregnant women. The baby, in utero, is a very sensitive receiver of energies and, as such, the healer needs to be careful not to push energy around strongly. Beginners do not realize how easily energy follows thought, and they may cause a disturbance to a fetus, especially in the first trimester.

In Lou's case, there were no known inherited factors for her thyroid imbalance, although her blood picture initially suggested Hashimoto's disease due to the presence of destructive antibodies; this thyroid problem is often an inherited tendency. As with the previous case, Lou is a very sensitive and intelligent young woman, and her thyroid was helped by the outer (naturopathic) and inner (esoteric healing) treatments. After an especially easy and beautiful birth experience (compared with her previous experience of childbirth), Lou felt especially well and her throat chakra remained in balance. The baby was placid and serene, which I often find happens after holistic treatment of the mother during pregnancy.

In summary, there is a relationship between the throat chakra, thyroid gland, throat tissues including the larynx and tonsils, and the lymphatic system, whose job is to cleanse all the body tissues. We have reviewed cases of lymphatic congestion from the less serious conditions of eczema, tonsillitis, and sinusitis, to more deep-seated lymphatic congestions of bronchitis and asthma, and serious conditions like lung cancer.

The throat chakra relates to our ability to express our innate creativity, and to feel free to express ourselves. Because of its connection with our mind, the throat chakra can condition our thyroid function through an overactive mind, either by producing busyness or worry. As with most parts of our body, the thyroid and respiratory organs can be affected by inherited factors. The case histories described have illustrated these points.

Healing Practice for the Throat Chakra and Chest Area

There are a number of triangles for this area: the lung triangle, diaphragm triangle, and the opening triangles. The chest triangle of force is also often used, which was described at the end of the previous chapter. The lung triangle strengthens the lungs and the diaphragm triangle is especially good for coughing, as it brings in the sedating effect from the vagus nerve. The opening triangles are especially suitable for bringing the energies of the throat chakra out through the arms, so that the person becomes more creative in a mental or physical way, or both. It is also good for those whose self-expression feels blocked.

1. Align as previously described. Place your hands on the client's shoulders and imagine linking up with your own soul, the client's soul, and the source of all healing and ask that healing take place according to the plan of the soul.

2. Visualize the healer's flow of energy by imagining the following alignment: soul, heart, head, and hands.

3. When you sense that the energies are flowing, move to the left-hand side of the client and kneel or sit so that you can comfortably have your hands on either side of their body. From this point on, you do not physically need to touch the client.

4. Balance all the chakras up the spine, as described earlier, by placing the right hand behind the spine of the client and the left hand in front. Sense the impact of the energies on the hands and move them gently in and out, in an accordion fashion, until the flow of energies seems balanced between your two hands. Balance the

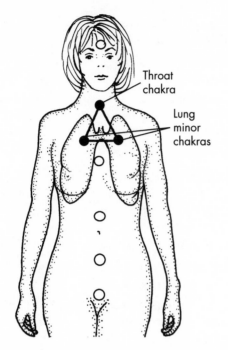

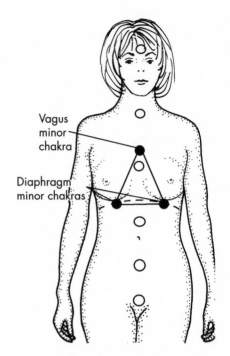

FIGURE 23: THE LUNG TRIANGLE. The lung triangle connects the throat chakra and lung minor chakras, and is vitalized for all respiratory conditions.

FIGURE 24: THE DIAPHRAGM TRIANGLE. The diaphragm triangle connects the vagus minor chakra, above the heart, with the two minor centers on the diaphragm.

chakras in the order of solar plexus, base, sacral, heart, and throat. During this process, there is no need to have the hands close to the body. It is best to have them as far away as possible, because it seems to be easier to assess the energies in this way and is less disturbing to the client.

5. Move some feet in front of your client to do the **lung triangle,** which consists of the throat center and the two lung points (see figure 23). In imagination connect, in thought, your brow chakra with the throat chakra of your client, and the hand chakras are connected with the lung minors of the client.

6. As with other triangles, do not be concerned about the exact position on your client of these minor lung centers because energy follows thought. So think of the three points, connect them with light, and then hold the triangles until energy flows.

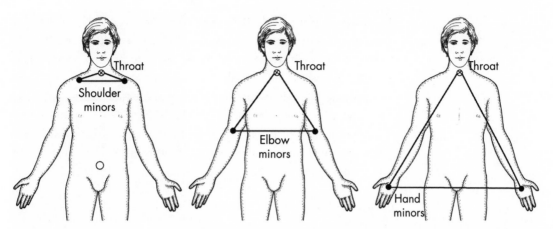

FIGURE 25: THE OPENING TRIANGLES. The opening triangles bring out the energies from the throat chakra and help our self-expression. They are visualized from the shoulder triangle downwards.

7. The **diaphragm triangle** comes next and involves the vagus center, just above the heart, and two points on the diaphragm (see figure 24). Connect, in thought, your brow chakra with the vagus center of the client and the two hand chakras with the diaphragm points on the client. Hold the triangle as above.

8. The three **opening triangles** consist of the throat chakra and shoulder minors, throat chakra and elbow minors, and throat chakra and hand minors (see figure 25). Imagine your brow chakra connected with the throat chakra of the client and then use the hand chakras to connect, in thought, with each set of minor chakras on the client: first the shoulder minors, then the elbow minors, and finally, the hand minors.

9. Connect the three points of light for each triangle and wait for the energies to flow before moving on to the next one. In this way, you gradually bring the energies down from the throat chakra and out through the arms, for the purpose of stimulating creativity and service in the client.

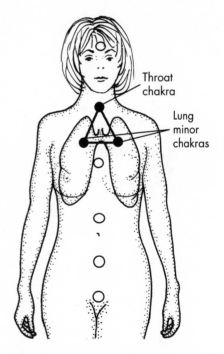

FIGURE 26: THE LYMPHATIC TRIANGLE. The lymphatic triangle connects the throat chakra with the lymphatic minor centers, situated at the center of each clavicle bone.

249

10. The actual **lymphatic drainage triangle** mentioned in some of the case histories is more difficult to describe, and would be best done with an instructor trained in esoteric healing. However, it would be useful for stimulating the lymphatic system to do the lymphatic triangle, which consists of the throat center and the two lymphatic minor chakras in the middle of the clavicles (see figure 26). Connect your brow chakra again with the throat and use the hand chakras to connect with the lymphatic points. Hold the three points, as usual, until sensing an energy flow.

11. Close as usual.

12 The Brow Chakra and the Nervous System

The brow chakra is involved in a synthesis or bringing together of all the facets in our personality and it, therefore, gathers up energies from all the chakras. It is appropriate that this is the final chakra to consider. The gland corresponding to the brow chakra is the pituitary, situated in the center of our head, behind the root of the nose. The pituitary has a relationship to all the glands related to the spinal chakras. Thus, we can see an analogy between the brow chakra and the pituitary gland, as both have a ruling effect over the other chakras and glands, respectively.

The pituitary gland is intimately related to a small body of nervous tissue situated near it, called the hypothalamus. The hypothalamus rules many nervous processes in the body. This is probably why I find its energy disturbed in most nervous complaints. It is always disturbed by worry and anxiety, and is often temporarily disturbed following menopause in women.

The minor chakras associated with the brow center are the eye minors and ear minors, and these are, obviously, associated with ear and eye problems, under the conditioning effect of the brow center. Other conditions covered in this chapter will include nervous disorders, such as tension and migraine headaches, nervous exhaustion, insomnia, palpitations, and multiple sclerosis.

The nervous stress of individuals in the twenty-first century is profound, but even as early as 1970, I found in my practice that nervous complaints topped the list of reasons clients visited my clinic. We need to constantly keep in mind the negative effects of mental and emotional stress on the nervous system via the chakras. Although the brow chakra is concerned with the nervous system, other chakras are also involved. For instance, emotional upsets that affect the nervous system will be related to energy coming from the solar plexus chakra, which is the gateway into our body from our emotional life. Mental worry and frustration will affect the nervous system via the throat chakra.

When considering the chain of energies that affect the nervous system, we have a flow connecting our thoughts, emotions, etheric body, nervous system, endocrine glands, blood, and tissues, in that order. So, apart from it being influenced by our thoughts and emotions, the nervous system can be influenced by blood that is deficient in those elements essential to it, such as the tissue salts magnesium and potassium phosphate and the vitamin B complex. These important nutrients may be deficient in the diet or they may become deficient due to an excess of nervous worry, whereby the nerves are constantly firing and using up these elements. A lot of study or long hours of work will have the same effect of depleting the system of elements needed for healthy nerve function.

You can see why we need to treat individuals with nervous problems holistically, so that the need for both supplements and the underlying cause for nervous stress are addressed. The esoteric healing helps balance the chakras, to remove underlying stresses, while the supplements strengthen the nervous system. In addition, I often teach a person meditation techniques (outlined in appendix 2), so that they can start each day relaxed but focused for work and challenges. Tai chi, yoga, and physical exercise are also ways for individuals to prevent and deal with tensions.

There are difficulties in this new century that have added considerably to our stress. One is the current work ethic, whereby an individual may stay in a work situation that creates enormous stress because they must fulfill huge financial commitments involving home mortgages, school fees, and desire for material assets, both for comfort and to keep up with peers. In many cases, there is a quite realistic fear that another job may not be obtainable, especially if the individual is over 40 years old.

It is inspiring that a growing minority embark on a spiritual journey to improve their nervous health by facing their fears and moving out of stressful work situations. Due to a new outlook on life, they attract suitable work. In other words, they have, in some way, aligned with their inner soul impulses, thus moving beyond personality restrictions and, in this new space, have caused an energy shift that has brought new opportunities into their life. This move takes courage, and involves the need for healthy energies flowing through the brow center, in keeping with control of the personality forces.

Another result from twenty-first-century busyness relates to children. Nervous stress and exhaustion in children often manifests because both parents are working and the children have to leave home very early each day and go to a child-care facility after school. So they have a very long day. My teacher clients tell me that many children in their classes have nervous exhaustion as a result. Their schoolwork then becomes poor, and there are more behavioral problems. Related to this process are the grandparents of children whose parents have separated and who are called upon to look after grandchildren several days per week. I have many exhausted grandparents as clients.

Conditions like insomnia, headaches, irritability, and nervous exhaustion are, therefore, endemic in the twenty-first century. Despite the labor-saving devices in modern living, the average person spends less time relaxing than ever before. I find in my meditation classes that most class members are unable to do meditation in the morning, because they must leave so early for work. When I ask them the reasons for attending my class in the first place, the universal answer is to obtain peace and serenity.

A major adjustment that the human nervous system has made in the last 100 years relates to environmental noise. A century ago, there was little noise on the roads except horses and carts and steam trains; there were no planes to disturb the skies. The worst aspect is that people are so used to noise today that they do not even hear it. I have had people tell me that they cannot sleep in a *quiet* location because they are so used to *noise*. It seems also that people are so noisy in their thoughts and emotions that it is disturbing for them to be in a quiet space, because they become more aware of their many disturbing emotions and thoughts, and feel uncomfortable. Have you heard teenagers say they can't study without having loud music in the background?

This assault of noise and busyness on our nervous system uses up minerals and vitamins, such as the vitamin B complex, at a much greater rate than in the days of our grandfathers, when life was more sedate. You can understand, therefore, why, in so many cases, we give magnesium phosphate to relax the nervous system and potassium phosphate to replace all the potassium that goes out of a nerve cell every time it fires during activity. Therefore, we use up more potassium when we are nervously stressed or assaulted by noise.

Another problem for today's nervous system is the accumulation of toxins from our food and the environment. Examples of toxic elements from the environment that can affect the nervous system are mercury (especially from dental fillings) and industrial chemicals, to which we are exposed or consume through processed foods. These build up in our tissues, including the nervous system. Toxins also are apparently generated by negative emotions and stress. These toxins from emotional causes are apparently released into the gut, and are as strong as any adverse toxins from the environment. You may recall, as an example, the unpleasant odor from the sweat of a person or animal that has been under nervous stress, indicating the affect of stress on our secretions.

Nervous Exhaustion

When treating holistically, it is difficult to put cases into easy categories. You may have noticed with my cases in this book that I am treating several conditions at once, but that these conditions are related. The next case of a young girl belongs to that kind, in which several conditions overlap; however, the main presenting symptom with Jessica was nervous exhaustion.

Nervous Exhaustion Case Study: Jessica, 14, was brought to my clinic because she was very tired all the time. She had undergone a blood test, which established that she was not anemic, but her diet was deficient in the elements necessary for healthy nerve function. She typically only had white toast for breakfast, white bread, cheese, and lettuce sandwiches for lunch, no fruit, and only vegetables plus lentil soup in the evening; she had twelve spoonfuls of white sugar daily in her tea, and indulged in chocolate.

Her iris indicated an acid build-up from consuming so much refined food, and the iris fibers were slightly wavy, indicating the need for calcium and magnesium. When checking her energy field, I found that all her chakras were undersized, indicating that there was insufficient energy flowing into her body from the chakras. As in most headache cases, the hypothalamus was disturbed; this is conditioned by the brow chakra.

Her naturopathic medicine regimen included colloidal sodium, calcium, and potassium phosphate, vitamin B complex, and vitamin C. The sodium helps calcium to be absorbed in an acidic body, and the potassium phosphate and vitamin B increase energy. In addition, she had our usual cleaning regimen of homeopathic liver and lymphatic toning drops. I explained the need for dietary changes and how her present diet contributed to the tiredness.

On her return visit, Jessica reported having had a fever for five days. From my viewpoint, this was an interesting sign, as the fever probably manifested coincident with her improved vitality, thus providing the means for metabolizing the toxins in her system. She had changed her diet to include wholemeal bread and had given up the sugar and chocolate. Her schoolteachers commented on the profound difference they had noticed in her energy.

Jessica stayed well and continued the basic naturopathic treatment. Small additions were made from time to time, such as vitamin B_2 when she had cracks at the corners of her mouth, and homeopathic hay fever drops during the spring. She received a healing for her energy field at each visit, and her chakras became normal in size. By the fourth month, she had increased her salad and fruit intake. She then had a bad bout of tonsillitis and lost ten pounds in a week.

The tonsillitis is another interesting sign because, as I've said, the tonsils are the gateway to the lymphatic system. From a naturopathic viewpoint, this episode could be considered as a retracing phenomenon. In Jessica's case, the retracing meant that her body energies had increased during the treatment period and there was then an automatic reaction to eliminate waste that had accumulated in the tissues over some years. The tonsils became involved because they are part of the lymphatic system. Tonsil infection indicated that waste had collected in the lymphatic system from the tissues. Without natural treatment during this period of tonsillitis, the accumulated toxins may have just stagnated in the lymphatic system. The treatment assists the waste to be eliminated through the normal channels of bowel, kidneys, skin, and lungs.

I advised her mother to purchase a high-strength echinacea supplement, the tissue salts ferrum phosphate and potassium chloride, and to increase Jessica's vitamin C intake. All these measures increase immunity and help to clear toxins in the lymphatic system. Jessica regained her weight easily after the tonsillitis, and has been very well ever since.

After seven months, we tapered off the treatment and she was then on a good diet. However, after a few months off treatment, she needed to go back on the herbs and minerals. Modern school life is very demanding, and naturopathic treatment can often be a valuable health insurance during the last years of grade school, when teenagers are under stress from school and rapid bodily growth. Jessica is a typical case of an adolescent who needed correction to her diet with supplements to make up for deficiencies from a poor diet over some years, and who needed esoteric healing to correct simple energy deficiencies resulting from stress.

As soon as the correct energies were supplied (including those in her diet), her body corrected its imbalances and she became well. Jessica's slight relapse indicated that these problems are not corrected overnight and can take many months, especially if the system continues to be under stress, such as occurs in the study years of a young person.

Tension Headaches

Headaches have always been a common ailment among patients coming to my clinic. These headaches are often described as throbbing and are classed as migraine headaches, even though a true migraine is a one-sided headache. Tension headaches usually result from a deficiency of the tissue salts magnesium and potassium phosphate; however, many headaches have their origin in a congested liver. Generally, I find that most headaches are a mixture of nervous depletion and liver congestion. A surprising number of teenagers suffer bad headaches, and this is obviously partly due to their study workload and, in some cases, to the expectations of their teachers and parents.

Tension Headache Case Study: Michelle, 13, was brought to me by her mother, suffering from headaches that lasted up to two days. She also had lethargy, a history of asthma, and was subject to viruses every eight weeks or so. Recently she had two hepatitis B immunizations. These immunizations could have caused liver congestion, and I found an energy disturbance in this area when doing the energy scan. The energy was also disturbed in her lymphatic system and brow chakra. In keeping with the energy scan, Michelle's iris showed an imbalance in the autonomic nervous system (related to the headaches) and some lymphatic congestion; this, together with the nervous imbalance, predisposed her to be asthmatic.

Generally, I find that most headaches are a mixture of nervous depletion and liver congestion. A surprising number of teenagers suffer bad headaches, and this is obviously partly due to their study workload and, in some cases, to the expectations of their teachers and parents.

Michelle's first prescription included colloidal calcium phosphate, for the asthma tendency, to strengthen the chest tissues, and help the nervous system. Michelle showed a zinc deficiency (she had many white spots on the fingernails), so this mineral was also given. I included homeopathic liver and lymphatic drops to tone the liver and cleanse the lymphatic system, and I gave her vitamin C (1 g, twice daily) for her immune system.

After one month, Michelle reported fewer headaches and asthma attacks, and her improvement continued over the next month. At the second visit, colloidal magnesium phosphate was added to further help the headaches. She continued to have fairly mild viruses, so I gave her a tablet containing colloidal iron phosphate and potassium chloride; over many months, the remedies continued to clear the lymphatic system of mucus, and her immunity began to improve. She developed acne, but it may have been due to the retracing phenomenon: as the chest improved, the body was healing itself from within outwards, so that some toxins manifested as acne. Homeopathic drops helped the acne, and I advised her to take vitamin E and a tablespoon of flaxseed oil daily to help the skin.

Her periods commenced and, as they were not regular, I added homeopathic drops to enable her cycle to become regular. The basic minerals were then tapered down to a maintenance dose, as headaches and asthma were no longer an issue. Her studies are becoming more demanding, so she is happy to stay on mineral treatment.

She has a regimen to undertake during viral attacks, which includes echinacea (3 g, three times daily), colloidal iron phosphate and potassium chloride (which covers the first two stages of infection—inflammation and mucus), and extra vitamin C as needed. But she rarely needs to implement this. Over the last few months, I have not bothered to do the esoteric healing, because she is well and she does not seem to need help in that direction.

Michelle is the opposite of the previous case, because I almost needed to discourage her from taking treatment after most of her problems were resolved. Her mother was a bit concerned that Michelle focused on her health problems too much. However, like many of my female patients in this age group, her periods tended to be quite unstable, even after the main treatment period was completed. This tendency of irregular menstrual periods that I have noted has increased over the last 20 years. I think it is an indication of increased stress in young people.

The main benefits Michelle gained from the treatment were the resolution of the headache tendency and a reduction of viral attacks. This provided her with the needed energy to face the most demanding years of her school life. If her periods become irregular again, she will, I trust, return for further treatment.

Second Headache Case Study: David, 26, a student of the visual arts, was a headache sufferer with lymphatic congestion, and had recently had a cold that lasted two months. As a child, he suffered night terrors and, more recently, had very anxious dreams. He had headaches throughout the week before visiting my clinic, and had just given up smoking. His diet was very poor, with white bread for breakfast and lunch, no salad, little fruit, plus meat and vegetables for dinner.

I assessed, through his iris, that David was very deficient in minerals, so his prescription included a mineral tablet with calcium, magnesium, potassium phosphate, zinc, and vitamin B complex; homeopathic liver and lymphatic drops for cleansing; and vitamin C. From an esoteric perspective, David had an energy disturbance in the hypothalamus, which is conditioned by the brow center; this related to the stress and anxiety he felt at night. The chakras were all inclined to be deficient in energy, which is unusual in a young person, unless the lifestyle is very poor. Esoteric healing included the chakra balancing, vitality triangles, lymphatic drainage for the sinus, and the sinus triangle (brow chakra and sinus points in the middle of the eyebrows); in addition, I used the clearing triangle (brow, heart, and solar plexus) to clear out old psychic debris and to help his anxieties (see practice at the end of this chapter).

On his return visit, David was having bad headaches with persistent sinusitis and nasal congestion and his hearing was affected, but he had improved his diet. I gave him a mixture of red clover, burdock, catmint, cat's claw for immunity, and skullcap for the persistent headaches. By the time of his third visit after another month, he was delighted to report improvement in all respects. His sleep, headaches, and sinus had improved and he had stayed on a good diet. His treatment was continued and the improvement was maintained.

I was surprised that David improved so quickly, but his improvement shows what can be achieved with a synthesis of treatment. All his symptoms—headaches, anxiety, and sinus problems—were closely connected with the brow center, but he needed the physical remedies to clean out lymphatic toxins and to make up for the mineral deficiencies. When he felt well, he asked to taper off treatment, but I suggested he keep on the mineral treatment for a bit longer, nine months in all.

Migraines

While tension headaches are often the result of a magnesium and vitamin B complex deficiency, I find that migraines often involve liver congestion. The diet can be imbalanced and the digestive system is weak as a result. Migraine sufferers are often worse after eating cheese, chocolate, or ice cream, because of the liver congestion. This is because the liver must supply enough healthy bile to emulsify the fats in order to make them digest easily. If the liver is congested, the fats are not digested adequately and can precipitate migraines and allergies to dairy products and chocolates. In treating migraines, as with most health disorders, I find it necessary to address the whole person. As you will see in the next case, there were many other health conditions to consider, so it was hard to know where to start.

Migraine Case Study: Kimberly, 37, had a history of very severe migraines that commenced at the age of 15. She also had a history of bronchitis, asthma, recurrent cystitis, hemorrhoids, herpes, hypogly-cemia, insomnia, and ovarian cysts.

Initially, she had treatment at age 27. At that time, I gave her col-loidal calcium and magnesium phosphate to balance her mineral sta-tus; colloidal ferrum phosphate and potassium chloride for her bronchial problems; a zinc salt and vitamin C for promoting immu-nity to prevent the herpes attacks; colloidal calcium fluoride for the hemorrhoids; and blood cleansing herbs and vitamin B complex for energy. Note that there were a lot of mineral deficiencies.

Later I gave her an herbal mixture, to regulate her hormones, which consisted of false unicorn root, chasteberry, motherwort, and Chinese angelica; even 1 ml of this mixture twice daily often allevi-ates hormonally related migraines. Treatment was continued, with a few variations in the remedies, for four months, after which there was considerable improvement in all areas.

However, four months was not long enough to deal definitively with her problems and, three years later, Kimberly came back for more treatment for ovarian cysts, psoriasis of the scalp, and hemor-rhoids. Her hormone drops were repeated, together with blood cleansing herbs for the scalp; colloidal sodium and calcium phos-phate for the skin and ovaries; zinc for immunity; and homeopathic drops for hemorrhoids. Once again, she did not have a long course of treatment.

When she returned some months later with bad migraines, I thought these must be connected with the ovaries because these organs had a disturbed energy pattern, according to my energy scan. This meant the headaches were probably hormonally based. Other symptoms included vomiting, muscular twitching, lost consciousness on many occasions, and she was having three attacks of these severe migraines per month. Her brow chakra, which governs the pituitary, which, in turn, regulates the ovaries, was disturbed.

I treated the headaches with colloidal magnesium and potassium phosphate; a small B complex tablet; an herbal tranquillizing tablet containing valerian, passiflora, skullcap, and hops; and liver and lym-phatic cleaning drops. I also prescribed a wild yam extract cream combined with chasteberry, homeopathic drops to balance the ovaries, and herbs to address the liver congestion (often associated with migraines). This herbal mixture contained dandelion, catmint, meadowsweet, centaury, and burdock. Colloidal calcium and sodium phosphate were recommended for her tendency to cysts in the ovaries.

I used esoteric healing on each of Kimberly's visits to balance the endocrine glands, using the endocrine pentagon. The nervous system was also balanced by using the vagus triangle (brow, alta major, and vagus center) and the grounding sequence. (The vagus triangle is described at the end of this chapter.)

After four months of treatment, Kimberly's migraines had completely gone. I am inclined to think today that a main factor in this resolution was the hormone-balancing cream plus the esoteric healing to balance the energies of the brow center, ovaries, and pituitary. It is always essential when faced with multiple problems, in such a case, to discern the main cause. It would have been easy to use an enormous number of remedies for all her ailments but easy, too, to have still missed the fact that the migraines were *hormonally based*, even though she had three per month.[54]

Kimberly has been with me as a client for a long time, and I consider her hormonal problems quite severe. The pituitary and ovarian disturbance has been responsible for her great difficulty in becoming pregnant, but with holistic treatment, she has now had two successful pregnancies; the second occurred after the headaches were resolved, when her body was in a balanced state and able to conceive. She is overjoyed, because it has taken six years since her first child to get pregnant again, although her natural treatment had some long breaks. Kimberly sees herself as a great worrier, and this, and her sharp intelligence, is in keeping with the potential of the brow chakra and pituitary gland to become energetically disturbed.

This case illustrates that we cannot consider the brow chakra in isolation from the sacral center (ovarian disturbance) and solar plexus (vomiting). As this case shows, there is always a complex intermingling of energy from one chakra to another, and this is why the treatment needs to be holistic.

Second Migraine Case Study: Gayle, 43, came for help with her optical migraines, associated with very low blood pressure. Optical migraine is a term meaning that the migraines affect the eyes; remember that the eyes are connected with the brow chakra. Gayle suffered occasional loss of sight with black patches in her visual field, and this obviously interfered with her ability to work and function. She had difficulty sleeping and was very tired. She had undergone a hysterectomy for fibroids four years ago. Her diet had included eight cups of coffee per day, but she had cut it down recently to three cups. Over the years, I have found coffee drinking to be very detrimental to migraine sufferers, because it causes a further imbalance in a nervous system already unbalanced. Gayle's iris indicated moderate toxins, fanning out from her digestive tract. From the energy scan I found her brow chakra, liver, and nervous system had energy disturbances.

Gayle had consulted me five years earlier for dizzy spells, tiredness, mood swings, and hypoglycemia, but her problems had resolved within four months, so she had discontinued treatment. However, she probably still needed more treatment then, for some of the basic imbalances of the digestive system that had led to the hypoglycemia.

For the current migraines, she received magnesium orotate, vitamin B$_6$, a digestive tablet with enzymes from papaya and other herbs, liver and lymph toning drops, and echinacea for her immune system. I also gave her subtle healing to balance her chakras and digestive system. I undertook particular work for the eyes, including triangles between the brow chakra and eye minors; eye minors, eye organs, and optic nerves; and the eyes. On her return visit in a month, she reported her headaches were less often and less severe, but as she was still very tired, her remedies were repeated.

It is not wise for those who have not worked under instruction from an esoteric healing teacher to work with the eyes, in case they cause an imbalance of energies, but I have included the first triangle of brow chakra and eye minors at the end of the chapter for your practice.

After another month, her energy had much improved and she had suffered only one bad migraine. I switched the magnesium orotate to magnesium and potassium phosphate, after which she only suffered one headache, and that was when she ran out of her homeopathic drops. I had put a neuralgia remedy called Spigelia in her drops from the first visit, and I think this helped her specific type of headache. Her improvement continued, with only occasional migraines, but these no longer produced any severe visual impairment and she reported that her digestion had also permanently improved.

This case was an interesting challenge, because the migraines were so severe. Again, I found a connection between the chakra and the associated organ, plus dietary indiscretions—coffee, in this case. Improvement manifested when the esoteric healing was combined with the mineral, herbal, and homeopathic supplements.

Apparent Psychosis from Mineral Deficiencies

Mineral deficiencies can sometimes have a dramatic effect, even resulting at times in apparent psychosis. I have had several clients who were labeled psychotic and prescribed antipsychotic drugs, which did not work or which they refused to take. These persons then became completely well on natural remedies. This shows the profound effect of minerals on the nervous system.

There seems to be a fine line between the states of exhaustion, tiredness, and more serious manifestations, such as paranoia and schizophrenia. There are, of course, also inherited predispositions towards schizophrenia, but these are understood by some psychiatrists as inherited biochemical inadequacies. Not all patients with these problems are prepared to take vitamin and mineral supplements, so compliance is very important. From the esoteric perspective, there is usually a problem with the brow chakra in cases of psychosis. It is usually overactive, and this correlates with the high intelligence of many schizophrenic persons.

Psychosis Case Study: Jo, 10, took his remedies and made an amazing recovery from apparent psychosis. He had been very anxious at school and was so paranoid about the furniture in his room that he could not go to sleep. He was on an antipsychotic drug, but it made him constipated, and his mother wanted an alternative. He also suffered a bit of asthma and his iris revealed lymphatic congestion. His diet was quite good, in that he ate whole foods. The supplements I gave him included colloidal magnesium and potassium phosphate, plus vitamin B complex for nerve balancing, a large dose of vitamin B_3 for the paranoia, and an herbal sedative tablet with valerian, skullcap, passiflora, and hops, taken before bed.

After one month, Jo was off his antipsychotic drugs and was much better, in terms of his paranoia, but as he still had troubles at night, I added homeopathic drops for sleep, plus the Bach flower essences Mimulus for fear and Hornbeam for strength of mind and body. These additions seemed to further settle him and help his sleep and well-being. After a few months, I added colloidal calcium phosphate to enhance his skeletal strength and address the asthma tendency, as well as homeopathic gland-balancing drops for his thyroid and testes. He had 18 months of treatment, after which he had no relapses of the panic attacks or paranoia.

Jo's case illustrates what can be achieved, with natural treatment, for a seriously unbalanced state of the nervous system and emotions. We could argue as to which came first, the nervous system severely depleted of necessary mineral salts or the fears that caused the nervous system to be depleted. Since we are talking about holistic treatment, this argument is irrelevant. By treating his nervous system with the mineral salts and vitamin B complex and B$_3$ and his emotional states with the Bach flowers, he made a complete recovery from the paranoia. Once a person is in a state of balance again, a good diet should maintain the improvement, provided there is no severe emotional stress or excessive need to study.

Nervous Tremor Case Study: Nervous problems often run in families. Jo's older brother, Alan, came to me some years later for help with nervous, shaking hands. An electrician by training, he needed to be able to do fine work with his hands. Alan also complained of poor concentration. He had a fairly poor lifestyle and was a regular smoker. Yet his shaking improved with just three items: a mineral tablet that included salts of magnesium, calcium, potassium, zinc, and large amounts of vitamin B complex; one gram of vitamin C, twice daily, to replace what was lost through smoking; and homeopathic drops for cleansing the liver and lymph glands.

After two months, Alan was able to give up smoking, and the shakes considerably diminished. He may not get rid of the tremor completely, but if he continues regular supplementation with the minerals, it should be minimized.

I thought the esoteric healing was important in a case like Alan's, because of the shock to his system from the discovery of his father's dead body. In discussion about this event, Alan said he was not shocked, because the family has been expecting the death for a long time. It seemed to me, however, that the shakes could well have developed in Alan as part of anticipatory anxiety that started years before his father's actual suicide, and that maybe he had underestimated the effect of this event on his nervous system. Perhaps he would have been better off to have manifested more anger and grief over the suicide and the shakes arose from the suppression of these emotions. The family had counseling at the time, but research on the results of trauma counseling leads me to believe its present form is not particularly helpful in most cases.

My healing approach for Alan was, therefore, to use the naturopathic treatment previously described, plus esoteric healing. After doing the chakra balancing and vitality triangles, I paid attention to his nervous system. That meant working with the alta major chakra at the base of the skull, plus the vagus triangle (brow chakra, alta major chakra, and vagus minor center) and the grounding sequence (already described; see appendix 1). The alta major center is situated in the area where the skull joins the spinal column and, therefore, is close to the medulla area of the brain. An emotional shock can affect the alta major center, which, in turn, affects the nervous system; a disturbance to the medulla could cause trembling of the hands.

Fortunately, Alan's shakes resolved considerably with the esoteric healing and the naturopathic medication. Perhaps, at some later time, he will wish to look deeper into the emotional situation but, at this point, he is not interested in going in this direction.

Loose Connection between the Physical and Etheric Bodies

I have described how the nervous system can be affected by a deficiency of minerals and vitamins in the diet on the one hand, and how these deficiencies can also be caused from an overworked nervous system resulting from emotional and mental stress. There is another more uncommon situation, whereby the nervous system is affected by lack of energy due to a loose connection with the underlying energy field called our etheric body.

You will remember that the etheric body is the energy field that interfaces between the astral or emotional and the physical body. For example, a general anesthetic pushes the etheric body out from the physical, and that is why we feel no pain when the surgery affects our nerves. Fortunately, we are prevented from dying because, with a good anesthetic, the much-reported "silver cord" that connects the etheric with the physical body remains unbroken. Likewise, in near-death experiences, the etheric is ejected, but if the silver cord were to be broken, the individual could not be revived.

Sometimes after general anesthesia, the etheric does not automatically become closely reknit with the physical body and the person is very tired and feels "woolly" in the head, because there is insufficient energy coming through the chakras into the physical nervous system. Esoteric healing and basic naturopathic treatment for the nervous system can be very helpful in these situations. The next case shows what a loose connection between the etheric body and the physical can generate.

Sometimes after general anesthesia, the etheric does not automatically become closely reknit with the physical body and the person is very tired and feels "woolly" in the head, because there is insufficient energy coming through the chakras into the physical nervous system. Esoteric healing and basic naturopathic treatment for the nervous system can be very helpful in these situations.

Loose Connection Case Study: Peter, 41, a building supervisor referred to me by his wife, needed treatment for tiredness, which was especially acute in the late afternoon. He complained of feeling very vague and experiencing taste distortions. He said he was worse at new and full moons; this probably related to the changes in the Earth's magnetic field at these times. His iris revealed a buildup of acidity and showed other toxins, in moderate amounts, in the gastrointestinal tract. At times, he craved salt or chocolate.

Peter reported having had a profound nervous disturbance earlier in his life, after having anesthesia. This effect was probably enhanced by the fact that he had taken recreational drugs earlier in his life, and he had a history of epilepsy as a young man. The tendency to epilepsy relates to a loose connection between the etheric body and the physical. The etheric scan made me aware of a gap between his etheric energy field and body. The energy flowing through the etheric chakras was short-circuited because of its separation from the spine, and the amount of energy was deficient. There was a weakness around the area of the brow and crown chakras that would have accounted for difficulty in concentration.

After the main chakra balancing, I paid attention to the vitality triangles and to connecting his energy field to the Earth, through the center below the navel (solar plexus minor center). The subtle healing was to strengthen the chakras and the connection between his etheric body and nervous system.

For the nervous system, I prescribed colloidal magnesium and potassium phosphate; vitamin B complex; the homeopathic liver and lymphatic cleansing drops; vitamin B_3 for the distortion of taste; and the Bach flower essences Mimulus for fear, Star of Bethlehem for shock, Clematis for vagueness, and Cerato for doubt.

Peter felt much improved within a month, and had more energy and less vagueness. The remedies were repeated for two months, and he showed consistent improvement. The salt craving continued into the second month so I gave him homeopathic salt in a high potency; after four doses at weekly intervals, this craving disappeared.

Peter then developed a rash on his legs that may have been part of the cleansing process, so I added an herbal tablet containing gallium and red clover to his prescription. Peter had to cancel his fourth monthly appointment due to working away from home, but his improvement apparently continued. Ideally, I would have preferred for him to continue the treatment for six months, as that is the average time needed for mineral deficiencies to be resolved. Individuals can often improve for a few months and then relapse, with further stress, if their treatment plan is shortened.

Insomnia

Insomnia can result from many causes, including mineral deficiency, anxiety, fear, other negative emotions, environmental noise, and hormonal factors. Women over fifty feature very strongly in this group of clients, and their sleeplessness often relates to a drop in ovarian hormone levels. From my studies, I would say that this drop in hormones affects the pineal gland, which has been shown to be the main regulator of our circadian or twenty-four-hour rhythm.

All of the chakras and their associated glands interact and affect each other. There is a feedback mechanism between the ovaries and the pineal, and possibly a drop in ovarian hormones will affect the pineal. The pineal gland is intimately connected with the body rhythms and is, therefore, one of the main regulators of our sleep. It secretes several hormones, including melatonin and serotonin, and these two hormones need to be in balance. Serotonin is necessary for relaxation and its production in the body is enhanced by the now famous herb, St. John's wort.

Other factors that effect the pineal gland are long flights across time zones and exposure to electromagnetic fields. Sleeping on an electric blanket or water bed or with your head too near a digital clock are factors that have been shown to effect the pineal gland.

However, there is also a close relationship between the pineal gland and the physical expression of the brow center—the pituitary. The pituitary is closely related to the nerve center in the brain called the hypothalamus, which mediates between the pineal and pituitary glands and the nervous system. I often find an energy disturbance in the hypothalamus in persons under nervous stress, and especially in women of menopausal age whose ovarian hormones are diminishing.

The main mineral salts for insomnia are those for all nervous problems—potassium and magnesium phosphate—as always, these should be taken in colloidal form. Other forms of magnesium such as chelates, orotates, or aspartates, can also be useful, but the practitioner needs to assess the cause of the insomnia. I have also found wild yam extract applied topically to the skin can regulate the ovarian hormones levels of the body, and that it is a lowering of these hormones at the time of menopause that causes insomnia in many women.

Insomnia Case Study: Rose, 52, had a bad case of insomnia. Since menopause, she rarely had more than two hours sleep per night. She also had pains in her left shoulder and suffered from hives. Rose was the main breadwinner, as her husband, who was ten years older, had retired. She had had a partial thyroidectomy (removal of thyroid tissue) for benign nodules ten years before, and her thyroid had been underactive ever since. Her diet was good and her iris revealed a good constitution, in terms of basic vitality, and a minimum of toxins, but it did show acute nerve rings.

I gave Rose the basic nerve tissue salts mentioned above—combined with vitamin B complex, homeopathic sleep drops, and an eye formula for sore eyes (she worked at a computer all day). She took these remedies for a number of months, after which her shoulder and hives resolved, but not her sleep problem.

An energy scan revealed that her chakras were deficient in energy and that the alta major center, in particular, was affected. The hypothalamus had disturbed energy. After the chakra balancing and the vitality triangles, I concentrated on the three head centers and their corresponding glands; I visualized a triangle between the pineal, pituitary, and carotid glands. This gland, related to the alta major center, is thought to relate to the fourth ventricle of the brain, but is not yet described in physiology texts (see chapter 4 for more on the alta major center). I also visualized a triangle between the anterior and posterior parts of the pituitary gland and the hypothalamus, and then did the vagus triangle for the nerves (brow/alta major and vagus center) and the grounding triangle sequence. Although I have not included all the head triangles in the practice exercises, I have presented the vagus triangle at the end of this chapter. Other head triangles should be studied with an instructor.

The esoteric healing on Rose seemed to have only a temporary beneficial effect on her sleep; basically, there was no improvement, and she would go to sleep at midnight and then be awake from 2 A.M. onwards. Then one day, in conversation, I found out that the main thing that seemed to be keeping her awake was worry over the situation of her young grandson. I immediately added Bach flowers to her prescription: Mimulus for fear, White Chestnut for persistent unwanted thoughts, Red Chestnut for worrying about other people, and Hornbeam for strength. The flower essences are wonderful for resolving negative emotions, and appear to work directly on the chakra system.

Rose began to sleep better immediately. She was able to go back to sleep again if she woke, and started to get five to seven hours sleep on a regular basis. Rose was ecstatic about this improvement and, occasionally, she even slept until 7 or 8 A.M.

Later, a complication arose. Rose relapsed to some extent, but still managed more sleep than before treatment. I suspect that her work practices affect her sleep due to the electromagnetic interference to her hypothalamus, pituitary, and pineal glands from wearing earphones all day. Thus, a combination of factors prevented Rose from sleeping: menopause changes in the hormones, worry at times over family situations, and electromagnetic stress from work that cannot be avoided because she must keep her job to pay the mortgage. The good result is that, at least, she is sleeping more than two hours per night now and she has times when she sleeps quite well.

Most clients improve their sleeping patterns after a few months on the tissue salts magnesium and potassium phosphate, but each case must be evaluated individually. The wild yam extract cream gives good results in many postmenopausal insomniac women.

Palpitations

Generally, with nervous problems, I find that there is need for attention to both the inner and outer requirements of the person, and that it is necessary to make an analysis of the predominant causes and then to make a synthesis of remedies to cover all the factors.

Palpitations Case Study: Paula had consulted another naturopath before me, so she was already familiar with naturopathic treatments. She was a 56-year-old schoolteacher who had suffered an aneurysm involving the brain twenty years earlier. She had kept fairly well since then, and was a vivacious woman who took her teaching work seriously and was in great demand as a substitute teacher. At the time she visited me, she was partially retired. Her main nervous complaints were palpitations and erratic blood pressure. Her iris fibers were slightly wavy; iridologists call this a neurogenic constitution, meaning it is subject to nervous complaints. This indicated the need for calcium and magnesium, the latter being the main remedy for palpitations.

Paula loved her regular monthly healing session with me, and felt serene and relaxed after each session. Her chakras were originally undersized due to tiredness, but became balanced during the treatments. Paula's history of blood pressure and the ruptured aneurysm suggested a disturbance of the brow center but, with palpitations, the heart chakra is also involved. So here again, we have a picture more complex than a disturbance in just one chakra.

The healing procedure, after balancing all the chakras and visualizing the vitality triangles, involved the vagus triangle to stabilize the nervous system (brow, alta major center, and vagus minor center) and the chest triangle of force (throat minors and breast minors) to strengthen the chest area. I did the grounding sequence to bring excess energies away from the head and down via the feet to the Earth (see the end of this chapter for vagus triangle and appendix 1 for the triangles previously described).

Paula's first prescription included colloidal calcium and magnesium phosphate three times daily, a small vitamin B complex tablet, and liver and lymphatic drops for general cleansing. She had no palpitations from that time onwards. After the second month, I added colloidal potassium phosphate to give her more energy. Her blood pressure stayed very stable for many months after treatment started, despite the fact that she took on more schoolwork for a term and with a very difficult class, which exhausted her. However, her palpitations did not return.

During this difficult period, she had a virus that caused laryngitis, for which I prescribed immune stimulating herbs, colloidal iron phosphate with potassium chloride, and extra vitamin C to clear the lymphatic system. She also complained of a knot in her chest, so I switched the magnesium phosphate to magnesium orotate, because it has more application to this type of problem; I also included homeopathic drops for her varicose veins.

Paula realized during the very stressful term of full-time teaching that it was not appropriate to put herself at risk in this way, and that it was not necessary, financially, to work full-time any more. Now she does the occasional relieving day here and there, and says she will not be pressured into larger commitments. I find that this is constantly an issue for clients, to find the right level of work and play for their health and financial needs. The most difficult pressures for clients to handle come from their families and peer groups. Thus, young people often feel they must push themselves to the limit, so as to have a better house, car, or more money to spend on luxuries.

In Paula's case, as with many others, the treatment phase provided both inner and outer sustenance, and appeared to give strength and space for reassessment of lifestyle and goals. Without the physical remedies for the nervous system, she may not have had the energy to think things through and the esoteric healing provided that link with her soul to touch the essence of her real needs.

Multiple Sclerosis

Perhaps one of the most serious and dreaded nervous system problems is multiple sclerosis (MS), in which the person gradually loses all control of their nervous system. Over the years I have treated people at all stages of this disease, and it has been mainly those in the early stages of the disorder who have persevered with the treatment. The problem often begins with tiredness and slight loss of coordination of legs or bladder, and progresses to possible death from lack of nerve transmission to the vital organs.

MS is an autoimmune disorder of unknown medical origin, but the effect is destruction by antibodies of the nerve coverings called the myelin sheath; it is this development that interferes with nerve transmission. Like other autoimmune disorders, such as lupus and rheumatoid arthritis, multiple sclerosis tends to affect young persons, often in their twenties, and they can end up bound to a wheelchair if the disease progresses.

Fortunately, in the following case, I was able to treat the person in the early stages of the disorder. It is an interesting case, because I was able to monitor progress over a ten-year period. MS is notorious for recurring from time to time but, nevertheless, I think that this case is a good illustration of the effective combination of natural therapies and esoteric healing.

Multiple Sclerosis Case Study: Lindsay came to visit me early in 1992, six months after being diagnosed with MS. He suffered a sensation of constriction around the waist, numbness in the fingers, and weakness in the legs. His symptoms had begun five years before, at age 23; he was 28 when he began naturopathic treatment with me. It was of interest that, as a young child, he was found to have a deficiency of white blood cells. This indicated that there was a possible problem with his immune system from an early age. Lindsay also has a history of mild asthma, and when I examined him, his energy was low. He has a busy job as a computer software specialist.

I was interested in the connection here between the brow center, mental work, the brain, and the loss of myelin tissue in the brain and around the nerves, which characterizes multiple sclerosis. Could a person with a tendency to excessive concentration (brow problem) develop a predisposition towards demyelinating their brain and nerves? Lindsay had a very cerebral job as a software engineer. His temperament, as a whole, was fairly intellectual, and he expressed little feeling. I often wondered if he thought the esoteric healing was just hocus-pocus. I wondered if, in the light of Lindsay's manifestation of an autoimmune disease, constant work with a computer and its associated electromagnetic field could be a factor in the destruction of his myelin within the brain and around the nerves.

From a physical viewpoint, the white matter, called myelin, around the brain connections and nerves has a great affinity with magnesium. Magnesium is commonly the most deficient mineral in the stressed nervous systems of modern humanity, and is especially indicated in multiple sclerosis.

Before his visit, Lindsay had been taking 500 mg of vitamin C and some vitamin E, and to these supplements I added a mineral compound containing the tissue salts calcium phosphate, magnesium phosphate, and potassium phosphate. The last two salts are the main "food" for the central nervous system, which is under assault in MS; the calcium strengthens the tissues. He was also given liver and lymphatic toning drops to cleanse the body of toxins, and lymphatic cleansing herbs such as burdock, poke root, clivers, and red clover. I added zinc to further assist the immune system.

Progress was slow, but over the next few months, there were slight improvements in energy and with the leg weakness; the numbness of the hands was slower to go. After a full year on the remedies, Lindsay showed consistent improvement. From time to time, I changed the herbs and gave him *pau d'arco*, a South American herb found to be effective in paralysis affecting the central nervous system in polio. This herb contains quinines, which are related to the electron system within the cell. This means the herb can increase the body energies overall by stimulating energy within the cell.

Over the next two years, Lindsay only had occasional relapses, which manifested as exhaustion; he also had leg aching or weakness. I gave him an extra remedy that released more oxygen for the muscles, and he stayed on this for a few years. This remedy was based on peroxides, which, in a suitable preparation, will have the effect of releasing more oxygen and hence, energy, into the tissues. It seemed to make a big difference to the energy available to his legs. This remedy was eventually unavailable, and we settled on another that released both hydrogen and oxygen in the body. The original research supporting this remedy included examination of glacial waters in areas where the populations were extraordinarily healthy into extreme old age. It was discovered that this water contained a considerable concentration of hydrogen and oxygen atoms and these were harnessed, in combination with homeopathic mineral salts, to provide a remedy that seems to energize all the cells of the body. Meanwhile, the basic minerals and the antioxidant vitamins C and E were continued, as were herbs for the immune system. By the middle of the 1990s, his improvement was stable and, during 1997, he remained well during an overseas trip.

By this time, I was combining the subtle healing with natural therapies for nearly all my clients and conducting an energy scan on everyone as part of my basic diagnostic. Lindsay had a relapse after a virus, which resulted in aching legs, and I discovered that the energy in his thymus gland was disturbed. It has often been observed that a virus can cause a relapse in an autoimmune disease, and this relates to my observation that the thymus gland was disturbed.

In addition, the energy in his brow center was excessive, compared to the energy in the other chakras, which seemed to correspond with problems of the nervous system. The healing sessions, therefore, included a balancing of all the chakras, the vitality triangles to improve his energy, the immune triangle (thymus and adrenal glands), and work with the brow and alta major centers and their corresponding glands. This involved making triangles between the three head centers (crown, brow, and alta major) and the three glands (pineal, pituitary, and carotid), then doing the grounding sequence to bring the energies down throughout the body. (As mentioned, the head triangles need to be learned under instruction, but see appendix 1 for a repetition of the other triangles.)

The healing session resolved this problem. Lindsay then went overseas and remained well, despite not taking any remedies, but a month after returning home, he had a bad relapse. His hearing was "woolly," the left side of his face was numb, and his sense of taste was diminishing. I found that the energy in his thymus gland was again disturbed and corrected this using esoteric healing. He regained his health quickly within a month.

After another few months Lindsay again went overseas to work. After returning, he had another relapse, with numbness of his left leg from hip to knee. It seemed to me that the long flight from London, after he experienced a cold winter, could have weakened his immune system. In keeping with this surmise, I found his thymus had again become disturbed. Since I did the subtle healing each time his thymus was disturbed, he made a quick recovery, whereas earlier, when I relied only on the remedies, his relapses lasted much longer.

Lindsay may have to stay on his supplements for many years, but compared to the alternative of progressing towards life in a wheelchair, I know he will not object. After fifteen years of symptoms, we would expect that his relapses might be worsening, but, in fact, he gets over such periods quicker than ever. Recently, he journeyed to Alaska and had no relapse with his health, and appears to be gaining stability of health all the time. It is now more than one year since I found any disturbances in his thymus gland.

This case illustrates clearly the benefit of using a synthesis of healing approaches. The esoteric healing was able to correct the disturbed energies underlying the immune system (thymus) and to remove any excess energy from the brow center (brain). The tissue salts for the nervous system were important to build up the mineral status and, hopefully, to provide the raw material for the myelin sheaths. Multiple sclerosis is known to have fairly long remissions but, in this case, Lindsay has remained well, on treatment, for ten years; the disease does not appear to be progressing, and he is nearly 40 years old.

A Case of Meniere's Syndrome: Medical problems with the pituitary and pineal glands are rare. However, I suspect that many subtle nervous disorders such as insomnia, relate to a disturbance of the pineal gland caused by electromagnetic fields. I often find some disturbance in the pituitary gland in the condition called Meniere's syndrome, which involves a disturbance in the inner ear and the semicircular canals. Symptoms include severe dizziness and, sometimes, vomiting. I always find that there is a nervous factor involved, and that good results are obtained using homeopathic drops and the mineral salts magnesium and potassium phosphate.

Charles, 51, is a business executive who does a lot of traveling each day to visit his clients. He collapsed a number of times, including once while driving, and was clinically diagnosed with Meniere's syndrome. On several occasions, when he collapsed, he was nearly unconscious. He has hearing aids in both ears, for deafness that occurred after a short exposure to extreme noise several years earlier. His diet is good, except for 28 spoonfuls of sugar in his tea every day.

On examination (and from intuition), I thought he was suffering more from severe nervous stress than from Meniere's. An energy scan revealed that both ear chakras were disturbed; these minor chakras are associated with the brow chakra.

His physical remedies included the mineral salts potassium and magnesium phosphate in colloidal form and vitamin B complex for the nervous system. He took chromium daily for his sugar craving, and sodium phosphate in colloidal form to antidote acid buildup in his tissues from consuming so much sugar. He took homeopathic drainage drops for his liver and lymphatic tissues to assist in detoxification and to drain off excess fluid from the ear. I gave him another homeopathic formula that included *Cocculus Indicus* (Indian cockleshell) as a specific for the dizziness associated with Meniere's syndrome.

In addition to the usual chakra balancing and vitality triangles, I used the following triangles: brow with ear minors; alta major with ear minors; the head triangle; the vagus triangle; the blood sugar triangle (pancreas and adrenal glands). I emphasized grounding energies via the traditional grounding triangles. (I mention these triangles for your general interest, but it is not advisable to undertake triangles on the head without detailed instruction from a teacher of esoteric healing. Several triangles involving the brow chakra are described at the end of this chapter.)

Charles has never had another collapse following vertigo since his first visit, despite the fact that his wife left him recently, an event that gave him a considerable shock. He has continued his treatment with me for over a year, and not only has he had relief from the Meniere's syndrome, but his sleep also has improved. He now only visits once every six weeks as we taper off treatment, and he has formed a new satisfactory romantic relationship.

Charles's case is significant, chiefly due to the connection between the brow chakra, alta major center, and nervous system, and, in this case especially, the effect of these chakras on the inner ears. The disturbance I found in the minor ear chakras may have been exacerbated by the electromagnetic effect from the wearing of large hearing aids in both ears. Although his case was medically assessed as Meniere's syndrome, it appeared that stress in the nervous system was the main cause for the vertigo and collapse; thus, the tissue salts for the nervous system were very important to correct deficiencies here.

During the treatment process, as so often happens, an underlying problem in his life surfaced and he had to reassess his situation, in terms of the most intimate relationship—the life partner. Charles made a big effort to find another suitable life partner. As the treatment progressed, the disturbance in the ear minor chakras completely disappeared. I think this resolved partly because of his psychological growth and partly because the mineral salts for the nervous system made him more resistant to other challenges, such as to the electromagnetic field from the hearing aids. So again, a synthesis of treatments produced the best results.

In this chapter, we have looked at the relationship between the brow chakra, the pituitary gland, and hypothalamus and some related nervous disorders. It is obvious that we cannot isolate these disorders to disturbances only of the brow chakra. For instance, in some nervous problems such as palpitations, the heart chakra or solar plexus are also involved, because our emotions are intimately related to the nervous system. Even in the headache cases we reviewed, the solar plexus was involved. This is especially the case in migraines, which have a relation to the digestive system and the liver. In the case of insomnia, we saw how Rose's sleep was sometimes affected by worrying about her grandson, how this worry related to the throat chakra, and that the associated fears were an expression of the solar plexus.

The synthesis of treatment in these cases shows the need for the outer treatment with minerals, vitamins, herbs and homeopathy to blend with esoteric treatment. In other words, there has been both inner and outer treatment for most of the cases. This has been a continuing theme throughout the book.

Healing Practice for the Brow Chakra and Associated Problems

The balancing for the brow center is different from that of the centers up the spine. Its entrance point is in front of the forehead, where we understand the brow center to be situated, but the exit point is not at the back of the head, as you might imagine in keeping with the spinal chakras. The exit point is a bit below and behind the top of the skull (see figure 27). We need to be very gentle when working on the head, and this is why the brow chakra is left until last to practice.

Hold your hands as in figure 27, keeping them well away from the head itself during the balancing. Use a gentle accordion motion for the balancing, as for the spinal chakras, so you can feel when the energy is balanced between the input on the forehead and the exit point. Now that you have learned how to balance the brow center, you can start each healing session with this center before the solar plexus.

In this practice session, we will do a triangle for the eyes, which can be used for any eye problems; the sinus triangle is for clearing the sinuses; and the clearing triangle, which connects the brow chakra, heart, and solar plexus, is for clearing old emotional debris, in particular, and the vagus triangle. The vagus triangle connects the brow chakra with the vagus minor center and the alta major center at the base of the skull; it is extremely useful for headaches, nervous tension, and pain.

1. Align as previously described: place your hands on the client's shoulders and imagine linking up with your own soul, the client's soul, and the source of all healing and ask that healing take place according to the plan of the soul.

2. Visualize the healer's flow of energy by imagining the following alignment—soul, heart, head, and hands.

3. When you sense that the energies are flowing, move to the left-hand side of the client and kneel or sit so that you can comfortably have your hands on either side of their body. From this point on, you do not physically need to touch the client.

4. Balance all the chakras and this time commence with the brow chakra, holding the hands as in figure 27.

5. Then balance the spinal chakras, as described earlier, by placing the right hand behind the spine of the client and the left hand in front.

6. Sense the impact of the energies on the hands and move them gently in and out, in an accordion fashion, until the flow of energies seems balanced between your two hands.

7. Balance the chakras in the order of brow (figure 27), solar plexus, base, sacral, heart, and throat. During this process, there is no need to have the hands close to the body. It is best to have them as far away as possible, because it seems to be easier to assess the energies in this way and is less disturbing to the client.

8. Now move several feet in front of the client and, in your imagination, connect your **brow chakra** with that of the client and your hand minor chakras to the **eye minors** at the outer corner of the client's eyes (see figure 28).

9. Gently allow the energies to flow through this triangle and when the flow is stable, in imagination, move your index fingers, which also contain minor chakras to connect, in imagination, with the **sinus points** in the middle of the eyebrows of the client (see figure 29). Again, wait until the energy is flowing freely through this triangle.

10. To do the **clearing triangle,** keep, by imagination, your brow chakra on the brow chakra of the client and connect, in imagination, one hand chakra with the heart chakra of the client and one with the solar plexus of the client (see figure 30).

11. Imagine the three points connected with light and wait until the energy is flowing. You might, to advantage, wait a few moments longer with this triangle than usual because, as mentioned above, it is a technique for eradicating old emotional patterns and debris, so as to clear the aura.

12. Now move to the left-hand side of your client to do the **vagus triangle.** In imagination, keep your brow chakra connected with the brow chakra of the client and place your right palm chakra about six inches under the base of the skull and your left hand about six inches away from the body of the client, just above their heart (see figure 31).

13. Connect these three points in light and then wait for the energy to flow. We do not usually teach this technique until part three

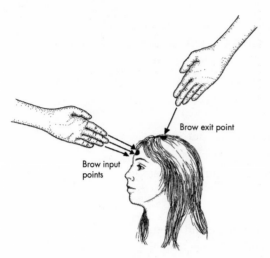

Brow exit point

Brow input points

FIGURE 27: BROW CHAKRA BALANCING. The hands should move very gently to balance the energies between the brow input and exit points. Hold the hands as far away from the head as possible, because the head energies are very sensitive.

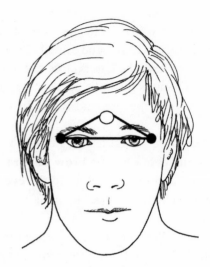

FIGURE 28: THE EYE TRIANGLE. The eye triangle connects the brow chakra with the eye minor chakras, located at the corner of the eyes.

of esoteric healing, but I am including this triangle in the book because there are so many nervous problems facing us today and it is a wonderful technique for calming the nervous system. Remember that all these healing procedures can be performed for friends and relatives at a distance.

14. As this is the final exercise, you can now learn to balance the three pairs of chakras. You may remember, we divided the chakras into three pairs in part one. The whole energy field is balanced before closing by balancing these pairs. The first pair to balance is the crown chakra and the base, which correspond to our will. We just use the two hand chakras for this procedure, so imagine one hand is above the crown and one below the spine. It is best to actually hold the hands well apart, so that one is above the other, to help the imagination along.

15. Keep the hands in this alignment and wait until there appears to be a balance of energy between the crown and base chakras of the client.

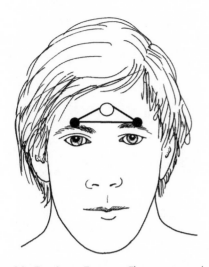

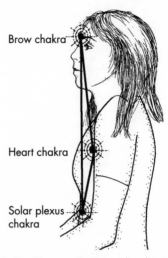

FIGURE 29: THE SINUS TRIANGLE. The sinus triangle connects the brow chakra with the sinus points, located on the center of the eyebrows.

FIGURE 30: THE CLEARING TRIANGLE. The clearing triangle connects the brow chakra, heart chakra, and solar plexus chakra. It is used particularly for cleansing the aura of old emotional issues.

16. Move the hands a bit closer together and imagine the throat chakra connected to the sacral center in the client and again wait until there is a balance of energies.

17. Finally, move the hands a bit closer together and visualize the hands connecting the heart chakra with the solar plexus chakra of the client.

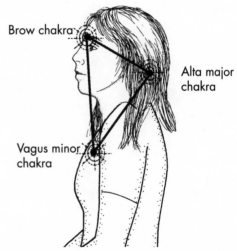

FIGURE 31: THE VAGUS TRIANGLE. The vagus triangle is used for all nervous complaints and consists of the brow chakra, the alta major center at the base of the skull, and the vagus minor center, situated above the heart.

Afterword

Healing is creative work. We can re-create our lives and bring all the parts together using many approaches, both inner and outer. In this book, I have attempted to describe how there are usually both inner and outer needs. This is why I find that combining the basic natural therapies of clinical nutrition, herbs, and homeopathy with esoteric healing to be generally successful. The inner healing seems to give the physical remedies a "kick start."

I often explain to my clients that once a physical condition has been established in the body, the underlying energy pattern becomes gradually distorted and does not always correct itself when the physical remedies, whether orthodox or naturopathic, are given.

One of the main problems with therapists of any kind results from a tendency to consider that one particular approach will cure everything. This applies whether the person is a medical doctor, a naturopath, herbalist, homeopath, masseur, or spiritual healer, to name but a few approaches.

In the past I used to get excellent results with about 70% of clients by using a synthesis of vitamins, minerals, herbs, and homeopathy, and I would never be tempted to give away these modalities. However, the results after adding the esoteric healing appear to be quicker and more thorough, and about 90% successful for those who are prepared to persevere for a few months or more. Since adding the inner healing for most clients, my practice has made another expansive leap, which, though I was not looking for it at this point in my career, has been a rewarding expansion.

There is an accelerating factor to consider in our healing adventures: the continuing speed and stress of the twenty-first century. The most consistent feedback I get after doing healing is the comment, "I could have gone to sleep" or "It made me feel so peaceful." People desperately need to relax and align with their inner essence so as to be able to cope with the many challenges they face. It is my hope that this book gives you ideas and practical suggestions for helping you to meet those challenges.

Summary of the Healing Practices

The exercises from each chapter have been gathered here in total for your convenience, so that you can see the full flow of exercises after having practiced each one separately. You should not attempt all the work here, but practice the triangles associated with each chakra, one at a time. This is to prevent energy overload. If you have not already done the practice with each chakra, start with the solar plexus, then work with the brow chakra after becoming familiar with the spinal chakras. The head energies are delicate; this is why you need to practice on the others first.

The triangles described for you to practice are by no means the only ones used by esoteric healers, but they will serve as a useful introduction for your first months of practice. Courses are available in most countries for those interested in further training.

Basic Protocol

Your basic protocol for a healing session is as follows:

Alignment: Place your hands on the client's shoulders and imagine linking up with your own soul, the client's soul, and the source of all healing and ask that healing take place according to the plan of the soul.

Visualize the healer's flow of energy by imagining the following alignment—soul, heart, head, and hands.

When you sense that the energies are flowing, move to the left-hand side of the client and kneel or sit so that you can comfortably have your hands on either side of their body.

Remember that the healing will be successful in proportion to *your* inner alignment with the soul. Daily meditation will be a great help to maintain alignment to your inner essence or soul and a suitable format is described in appendix 2. Also, by doing some kind of alignment or centering on a daily basis, the alignment process with a client during a healing is enhanced.

You can work on a client who is physically present or absent, or on yourself. If you are working on yourself, you simply imagine during the healing that your etheric body is sitting in front of you, and you carry out the same procedure as if there was a physical body of another person on the chair. The same process can be used when healing another person at a distance. Alternatively, when healing yourself, imagine your energy body is sitting sideways on your lap for the chakra balancing and then turn this energy body around to face you when doing the triangles.

Balancing Brow and Spinal Chakras: Assuming that you have already done some practice, you may start with the brow as follows. The balancing for the brow center is different from that of the centers up the spine. Its entrance point is in front of the forehead, where we understand the brow center to be situated, but the exit point is not at the back of the head as you might imagine, in keeping with the spinal chakras. The exit point is a bit below and behind the top of the skull (see figure 27). We need to be very gentle when working on the head, and this is why the brow chakra is left until last to practice.

Hold your hands as in figure 27, keeping them well away from the head itself during the balancing. Use a gentle accordion motion for the balancing, as for the spinal chakras, so that you can feel when the energy is balanced between the input on the forehead and the exit point. Now that you have learned how to balance the brow center, you can start each healing session with this center before the solar plexus.

Balance all the chakras up the spine, as described earlier, by placing the right hand behind the spine of the client and the left hand in front.

Sense the impact of the energies on the hands and move them gently in and out, in an accordion fashion, until the flow of energies seems balanced between your two hands.

Balance the chakras in the order of solar plexus, base, sacral, heart, and throat. During this process, there is no need to have the hands close to the body. It is best to have them as far away as possible, because it seems to be easier to assess the energies in this way and is less disturbing to the client.

Vitality Triangles: You can now start to practice triangles that will help to energize the body. These energies involve the base chakra, adrenal minors, spleen chakra, sacral chakra, and throat chakra. Have a look at the diagrams of the vitality triangles and adrenal triangle before and during the exercise when necessary.

First, do the *spleen triangle*, which is one of the vitality triangles, which brings in energy to the body. This triangle is comprised of the spleen chakra, spleen organ, and solar plexus (see figure 14).

Stand a few feet in front of the client.

Connect, in imagination, your brow chakra with the solar plexus, and imagine connecting one hand chakra with the spleen chakra and one with the spleen organ itself.

Visualize lines of light connecting these three points and wait a few moments until you sense the energy is flowing.

We now move to the *lower vitality triangle*, which involves the base, sacral, and spleen chakras (see figure 15).

Connect, in imagination, your brow chakra with the base chakra, one hand chakra with the sacral chakra and the other with the spleen.

Connect the three points with light and wait a few minutes until you sense that the energy is flowing freely.

Then make the *lower pranic triangle* by simply moving the right hand off the spleen and up to the throat chakra. The brow chakra stays connected with the base and the left hand with the sacral center. So the three points of the lower pranic triangle are the base, sacral, and throat chakras (see figure 16).

As before, hold these points for a few moments and sense the energy flow.

Choose the Chakra and Organ System Needing Attention: According to what you noticed during the chakra system, and also in keeping with the problems discussed with the client, you will now choose to work with a particular area or areas. If there are reproductive problems, you will work with the sacral triangle and endocrine

Chart of Triangles for

Base or Root Chakra for Energy, Kidneys, Ureters, Spine, and External Genitalia

Adrenal Triangle: Base chakra + adrenal minor chakras (figure 13)

Lower Vitality Triangle: Base chakra + sacral + spleen (figure 15)

Lower Pranic Triangle: Base chakra + sacral + throat (figure 16)

Further Vitality Triangles

Spleen Triangle: Spleen chakra + spleen organ + solar plexus (figure 14)

Pranic Triangle: Spleen chakra + minor chakra above heart + minor chakra below heart (figure 5)

Sacral Chakra, Reproductive Triangles, and Endocrine Balancing

Sacral Triangle: Sacral chakra + ovarian minor chakras or testicular minor chakras (figure 8b)

Grounding Triangles: Sacral chakra + hip minors, sacral chakra + knee minors, sacral chakra + feet minors (figure 8c)

Endocrine Pentagon: Pituitary gland + adrenal minors + ovarian or testicular minors (figure 19)

Solar Plexus Chakra and Triangles for Stomach, Liver, Pancreas, and Small Intestine

Liver Triangle: Solar Plexus + + liver minor chakra (figure 1

Stomach Triangle: Solar Plex stomach + stomach minor ch (figure 11)

Digestive Organ Triangle: Liv stomach + pancreas (figure 1

pentagon with, perhaps, the need for the lymphatic triangle to be energized for cleansing purposes. If there are digestive problems, you will work with the digestive triangles, and so on.

Balancing the Pairs: We balance them from without inwards, and this technique is used so that, after doing the various healing procedures, the whole energy field is balanced before closing. The first pair to balance is the crown chakra and the base, which correspond to our will. We use the two hand chakras for this procedure and imagine one hand is above the crown and one below the spine. It is best to actually hold the hands well apart, so that one is above the other, to help the imagination along.

Keep the hands in this alignment and wait until there appears to be a balance of energy between the crown and base of the client.

Each Body System and Chakra

Chakra, Blood Pressure, ...mune Triangle	Throat Chakra, Lymphatic System, and Opening Triangles	Brow Chakra and Nervous System Triangles
...e Triangle: Thymus gland + ...al minors (figure 20)	Opening Triangles: Throat chakra + shoulder minor chakras, throat chakra + elbow minor chakras, throat chakra + hand minor chakras (figure 25)	Eye Triangle: Brow chakra + eye minor chakras (figure 28)
...Triangle of Force: Throat ...chakra + breast minors ...ce breast minors with heart ...d throat chakra with throat ...below throat) (figure 21)	Lung Triangle: Throat chakra + lung minors (figure 23)	Sinus Triangle: Brow chakra + sinus points (center of eyebrows) (figure 29)
...Pressure Triangle: Brow ... + heart chakra + spleen ... (figure 22)	Diaphragm Triangle: Vagus minor + diaphragm points (figure 24)	Clearing Triangle: Brow chakra + heart chakra + solar plexus chakra (figure 30)
	Lymphatic Triangle: Throat chakra + lymphatic minors (center of clavicles) (figure 26)	Vagus Triangle: Brow chakra + vagus minor chakra + alta major (base of skull) (figure 31)

Move the hands a bit closer together and imagine the throat chakra connected to the sacral center in the client and, again, wait until there is a balance of energies.

Move the hands a bit closer together and visualize the hands connecting the heart chakra with the solar plexus chakra of the client.

Closing: Close the aura of the client by using the hands or imagination to make the shape of an aura around the client, from the feet upwards, with a gentle sweeping motion.

Imagine gently withdrawing the healing energy back through the hands to your soul, so as to break the connection with the client now that the healing is completed.

Visualize closing up your own aura in whatever way seems best.

To do this, you can imagine using the same movement on yourself as has been used for the client.

If you are working on yourself rather than with a client, you simply imagine that your etheric body is sitting in front of you and you carry out the same procedure as if there was a physical body of another person on the chair. Alternatively, you, the healer, can imagine that your energy body is sitting sideways on your lap for the chakra balancing and then turn this energy body around to face you when doing the digestive triangles. The same process can be used when healing another person at a distance.

Triangles and Procedure for Each Body System and Chakra

THE SACRAL CHAKRA AND REPRODUCTIVE SYSTEM: Use these exercises for any problems involving the uterus, ovaries, fertility, sex, prostate gland, or in a psychological sense, the handling of money. Physical problems may include ovarian cysts, irregular periods, endometriosis, pelvic pain, prostatic enlargement, or infertility in either sex.

The focus is on the sacral chakra and the triangles associated with the minor chakras related to this chakra—the gonadal, hip, knee, and foot minors. The endocrine pentagon—pituitary gland, adrenal glands, and ovaries or testes—is also often used to regulate the hormones. The lymphatic triangle (see page 293) could also be used for pelvic congestions.

The Sacral Triangle: Stand a few feet in front of the client and visualize connecting the brow chakra to the sacral center, which is situated just above the pubic bone.

Imagine connecting the left hand chakra to the right ovary minor chakra of the client (on your left) and the right hand to their left ovary minor chakra (see figure 8b).

Imagine lines of light between these three points and hold the points until you sense the energy is flowing freely.

Make a triangle, in imagination, between the ovaries themselves and the uterus and imagine tracing these organs in light. In the case of males, you will be making the triangle between the sacral center and the minors associated with the testes.

The Grounding Triangles: To do the grounding triangles, keep your brow chakra focused on the sacral center and visualize triangles between the sacral center and hip minors, then sacral center and knee minors and, finally, sacral center and foot minors (see figure 8c).

Wait while doing each triangle until the energy seems to be flowing. The purpose of these triangles is to ground energy that has been accumulating excessively, not only in the sacral center, but also in the whole body or, to psychologically "ground" someone who needs to be more practical by developing the ability to materialize their ideals.

The Endocrine Pentagon: The endocrine pentagon is used for balancing the hormones in cases of premenstrual tension, irregular periods, postmenopause problems, and infertility (see figure 19). There are five points here, as the name suggests. Place your brow center, in imagination, on the brow center of the client, and place your hands so that one hand chakra points to the adrenal gland and ovary on one side of the client and the other hand addresses the other adrenal gland and ovary. Remember that energy follows thought, and it is mainly our thought in the healing process that counts in these relationships between the healer and the client.

THE SOLAR PLEXUS CHAKRA AND THE DIGESTIVE SYSTEM: Exercises here will be useful for all digestive problems, such as indigestion, constipation, diarrhea, hepatitis, pancreatitis, diabetes, gallstones, stomach ulcers, and cancer of the digestive area. We also focus on the solar plexus and digestive triangles when emotional upsets have affected the digestive system.

Liver Triangle: Now move in front of the client and, from a distance of a few feet, imagine connecting your brow chakra with the solar plexus of the client and connect, in imagination, your palm chakras with the liver and liver minor center (see figure 10).

Do not worry about the exact position of the liver minor—remember that energy follows thought and just think "liver minor" and the energy will flow to the right place.

Imagine connecting the three points of solar plexus, liver organ, and liver minor center with light, then visualize the whole triangle to be filled with light.

Wait a few moments until the energy is stabilized.

Stomach Triangle: Now make a second triangle by keeping the brow center focused on the solar plexus and use the palm chakras to connect with the stomach and stomach minor chakra.

Visualize three points of solar plexus, stomach organ, and stomach minor as connected by a triangle of light and then fill the whole triangle with light (see figure 11). You do not need to see the lines of light in a physical sense, as it is sufficient to imagine the quality of light linking the three points.

Digestive Organ Triangle: The third triangle connects the three digestive organs of pancreas, liver, and stomach. So move your brow center to focus on the pancreas while one palm center connects with the liver of the client and the other palm center with the client's stomach (see figure 12).

THROAT CHAKRA AND THE RESPIRATORY SYSTEM: These triangles are vitalized for any respiratory problems, such as asthma, bronchitis, tonsillitis, laryngitis, or thyroid problems. The opening triangles are useful for bringing out the creative energy of the client and for self-expression. For respiratory problems, it is a good idea to do all the triangles in this section. The chest triangle of force is described below, under the section on the heart and is also useful for all respiratory conditions.

Lung Triangle: Move some feet in front of your client to do the lung triangle, which consists of the throat center and the two lung points (see figure 23).

In imagination, connect your brow chakra with the throat chakra of your client and the hand chakras are connected, in thought, with the lung minors of the client.

As with other triangles, do not be concerned about the exact position on your client of these minor lung centers, because energy follows thought. So think of the three points, connect them with light, and then hold the triangles until energy flows.

Diaphragm Triangle: The diaphragm triangle comes next, and involves the vagus center, just above the heart, and two points on the diaphragm (see figure 24).

Connect, in thought, your brow chakra, in imagination, with the vagus center of the client and the two hand chakras with the diaphragm points on the client.

As usual, connect the three points in light and wait for the energy to flow. This is a good triangle for calming down a continual cough.

Opening Triangles: The three opening triangles consist of the throat chakra and shoulder minors, throat chakra, and elbow minors, and throat chakra and hand minors (see figure 25).

Imagine your brow chakra connected with the throat chakra of the client and then use the hand chakras to connect with each set of minor chakras on the client—first the shoulder minors, then the elbow minors and, finally, the hand minors.

Connect the three points of light for each triangle and wait for the energies to flow before moving on to the next one. In this way, you are gradually bringing the energies down from the throat chakra and out through the arms, for the purpose of stimulating creativity and service in the client.

Lymphatic Triangle: The actual lymphatic drainage mentioned in some of the case histories is more difficult to describe, and would be best done with an instructor trained in esoteric healing. However, it would be useful for stimulating the lymphatic system to do the lymphatic triangle, which consists of the throat center and the two lymphatic minor chakras in the middle of the clavicles (see figure 26).

Connect your brow chakra again with the throat and use the hand chakras to connect with the lymphatic points. Hold the three points, as usual, until sensing an energy flow.

Heart Chakra, Circulatory and Immune System: The practice under this section is useful for all heart problems, whether physical or psychological. Physical disorders might include palpitations, irregular heart beat, low or high blood pressure, and poor immunity, or psychological problems like grief or sadness.

The Immune Triangle: Move a few feet in front of the client and connect your brow chakra, in imagination, to the thymus gland, situated just above the heart, and the hand chakras, one to each adrenal gland, situated just above the kidneys. Connect the three points with light and wait until the energy flows. This exercise stimulates and balances the thymus gland and adrenal glands in a way that also balances and stimulates the immune system (see figure 20).

The Chest Triangle of Force: The chest triangle of force is useful for strengthening all structures within the chest cavity, including the heart and thymus gland.

Use the hand chakras to balance between the throat center and the throat minor center just below it. So this is a straight line, rather than a triangle.

Hold these two points, in imagination, with the hand chakras until you sense a balance between them.

Connect, in imagination, your brow chakra with the heart chakra of the client, connect the hand chakras with the breast minors, and then connect these three points with light.

Wait, as usual, until the energy is flowing (see figure 21).

The actual triangle of force is then vitalized by keeping your brow chakra connected with the client's throat chakra, using the hand chakras to connect, in imagination, one with each breast minor. (The breast minors are just above the nipples as in figure 20.) Connect the three points—throat minor and breast minors—in light and wait for the energy to flow.

Blood Pressure Triangle: To vitalize the blood pressure triangle, you will connect the following points in the client—brow chakra, heart chakra, and spleen chakra.

Connect, in imagination, your brow chakra with that of the client and use one hand chakra to connect, in imagination, with the heart chakra of the client and the other to connect with the spleen chakra.

Visualize these points to be connected by light.

Wait, as usual, until the energies are flowing between the three points (see figure 22).

THE BROW CHAKRA AND THE NERVOUS SYSTEM: The brow chakra practice includes work for the eyes and sinuses, and this brings in the eye minors and the sinus points. We can do a triangle between the brow chakra and eyes for eye problems, and the sinus triangle between the brow chakra and sinus points on the eyebrows for clearing the sinuses. The clearing triangle connects the brow chakra, heart, and solar plexus for clearing old emotional debris, in particular. The vagus triangle also involves the brow chakra, in a triangle with the vagus minor center above the heart and the alta major center at the base of the skull, and is extremely useful for headaches, nervous tension, and for pain.

The Eye Triangle: For the eye triangle, move several feet in front of the client and, in your imagination, connect your brow chakra with that of the client and your hand minor chakras to the eye minors at the outer corner of the client's eyes. Gently allow the energies to flow through this triangle until the flow is stable (see figure 28).

The Sinus Triangle: Keep your brow chakra, via imagination, connected to that of the client and use the tiny chakras on your index fingers to connect with the sinus points in the middle of the eyebrows of the client. Again, wait until the energy is flowing freely through this triangle (see figure 29).

The Clearing Triangle: To do the clearing triangle, keep your brow chakra on the brow chakra of the client and connect, in imagination, one hand chakra with the heart chakra of the client and one with their solar plexus (see figure 30).

Imagine the three points as connected with light and wait until the energy is flowing.

Wait a few moments longer with this triangle than usual because, as mentioned above, it is a technique for eradicating old emotional patterns and debris, so as to clear the aura.

The Vagus Triangle: Now move to the left-hand side of your client to do the vagus triangle.

In imagination, keep your brow chakra connected with the brow chakra of the client and place your right palm chakra about six inches under the base of the skull (alta major center) and your left hand about six inches away from the body of the client, just above their heart (vagus minor).

Connect these three points in light and then wait for the energy to flow (see figure 31). We do not usually teach this technique until part three of esoteric healing, but I am including this triangle in the book because there are so many nervous problems facing us today. It is a wonderful technique for calming the nervous system.

The Base Chakra and the Urinary System: The base chakra features in the lower vitality and lower pranic triangles, and these have been described above under the protocol. If the base energy is found to be low, it is a good idea to add the adrenal triangle to the vitality triangles.

Adrenal Triangle: Stand a few feet behind the client and imagine connecting your brow chakra to the base center and also connect the hand chakras, in thought, with the adrenal minors. As before, do not be too concerned whether you are visualizing the minor chakras in exactly the right place above the kidneys. Remember that energy follows thought and after connecting the three points, visualize lines of light between the three points. Wait a few moments, until you have a sense of energy flowing freely through this triangle. This triangle is called the adrenal triangle (see figure 13).

Introduction to Meditation

Alignment

(Corresponds with inhalation.)

Visualize sitting in front of the sea early in the morning, just as the sun is rising over the water. The surface of the water is calm and still, reflecting the rays of the sun, which symbolize spiritual energies in the universe radiating towards us. Follow a threefold alignment:

Physical: Move the awareness around into all areas of stress. Visualize the rays of light irradiating all parts of the body, from toes to top of the head. Then become aware of the breathing rhythm, and quietly visualize energy flowing in and out with each breath, connecting us to all parts of the universe.

Astral: Become aware of the astral or feeling nature. Imagine all negative emotions flowing out into the sea; dissolving away and becoming transmuted by the rays of the sun. Experience the astral/feeling nature as translucent and serene—like a crystal clear pool.

Mental: Move back onto a high hill overlooking the sea. This hill symbolizes the mind, able to see life from many directions or viewpoints. As thoughts arise in the mind, imagine them as small fluffy clouds and allow them to drop off the side of the hill into space, leaving the mind quiet and focused.

Briefly visualize the threefold physical, astral, and mental nature as being aligned and free of all blockages, so that healing spiritual energies can flow through the personality.

Higher Interlude

(Corresponds to the pause between inhalation and exhalation.)

This is a time for quiet reflection and contemplation, with the consciousness centered in our inner Self or soul. Fly like a bird from the hill of mind into the inner soul or essence, and allow the personality self to become receptive to the healing energies of our inner Being.

A seed thought can be used here. For example, "I build a lighted house and therein dwell." Explore this concept from many angles, with the mind both in an individual and global sense, then when no further ideas can be explored, maintain the alignment and allow the inner energies to flow. (This stage can vary from 3–10 minutes in duration.)

Precipitation

Visualize the qualities received as golden and rose-colored healing energies, flowing in ever-widening circles to include family and associates, and also to vitalize new projects. See the energies flowing down and clarifying the mind, stabilizing the astral nature, and strengthening the etheric/physical nature.

Lower Interlude

(Corresponds to the pause between exhalation and inhalation.)

Take a few minutes to plan the work for the next 24 hours, so as to best keep the inner alignment or balance. Visualize a rainbow bridge of light and love, spanning the next 24 hours—imagine walking on that bridge throughout the day and night, radiating light, love, and the will to do good.

Reprinted from *Meditation the Most Natural Therapy* by Judy Jacka, Lothian Books, Melbourne.

Nutritional Suggestions

Clients are often confused as to what constitutes a good diet. Books and journals give conflicting advice, and individuals often wonder if they need a particular diet for a specific ailment. With the recent emphasis in the media on allergies, the challenge of a suitable menu for each individual has increased.

We each have an individual biochemistry, so no one regimen is suitable for everyone. It is the aim of the natural therapist to help restore the client to health, so that their digestive organs will cope with a wide range of whole foods. It is preferable to take the view that allergies result from an imbalance within our biochemistry and physiology that can be corrected, rather than to restrict the diet to a narrow range of items, which, in turn, restricts the social life.

Modern food processing and twenty-first-century living expose us to an ever-increasing range of chemicals that affect our food chains, drinking water, and air. This exposure presents our bodies with difficult challenges at times. Nevertheless, despite chemical assaults, a diet consisting largely of salads, fresh vegetables, whole grains, nuts and seeds, with the addition of small amounts of fish, chicken, meat, or other vegetarian protein can keep us in good health. So do not allow fears of environmental pollution to discourage you from selecting food in its natural state, preferably seeking supplies from organic food outlets.

The following points are general suggestions:

1. Select food that is as close as possible to its natural state. This means that packaged, tinned, refined, colored, flavored, pickled,

salted, and artificially sweetened foods should be kept to a minimum.

2. Proteins such as pasteurized milk, and items such as meat, cheese, and eggs should only be consumed in moderate amounts, because excess protein can cause putrefaction in the colon. In addition, undigested protein molecules can pass through the gut wall, causing allergies. Cow's milk should be limited to 250 ml per day for both children and adults and calcium obtained from others sources, such as almonds, sesame seeds, leafy greens, and dates. Many individuals cannot digest cow's milk, and it can contribute to eczema, asthma, and hay fever. Substitute beverages may include soy milk, goat's milk, rice milk, and fruit juices, preferably fresh or in glass bottles.

3. Start the day with fruit that is in season, as this is less likely to be from cold storage. The effect of fruit on an empty stomach stimulates the digestive enzymes and prepares the digestion for the day's work. This regime in itself can improve a sluggish bowel. It is also good to have some raw food with every meal.

4. Use whole grain cereals such as unpolished rice, millet, rolled oats, buckwheat, or barley. Include vegetable proteins such as chick peas, lentils, brown beans, soybeans, and use a variety of wholemeal breads such as wheat, spelt wheat, or rye. As we tend to eat far too much wheat, it is often preferable to eat breads from whole grain cereals, apart from wheat. Use wholemeal pastas and do not fall into the trap of eliminating three or four vegetables from the evening meal due to an emphasis on pasta. Meusli is not a particularly good way to have cereal, as we obtain more benefit from cooked grains. It is of value to include a selection of nuts and seeds in the diet, but they should be fresh, so as to contain oils that have not become rancid.

5. To keep your cholesterol in balance, you need far more omega-3 fats than are present in the average diet. The best source is flaxseed oil; 1-2 tablespoons should be consumed daily, and can be taken with lemon juice as a salad dressing, on cereal, or sim-

ply by the spoon. It should be kept refrigerated and never used in cooking. Olive oil should also be consumed in dressings on salad, as it provides a good balance for the flaxseed oil. Food should not be cooked in oils, as they are spoilt in the cooking process. It is preferable to pan fry in small amounts of butter.

6. Beverages should include 6–8 glasses of water daily, herbal teas such as peppermint, chamomile, or fennel, cereal coffees, or green tea. Both coffee and ordinary tea are dehydrating, and coffee unbalances the nervous system and is especially contraindicated in headache sufferers or individuals suffering from hypoglycemia. Alcohol should be limited to one or two glasses of wine or equivalent beverage daily.

7. Cooking utensils should be stainless steel, glass, or enamel.

Foods to Avoid	**Foods to Include**
White sugar products	Honey
White flour products	Millet, oats, buckwheat, barley, rice
Refined salt	Sea or vegetable salt
Biscuits, cakes, and pastries made with white sugar, flour, and preservatives	Wholemeal bread and cakes
Cordials and aerated drinks	Fresh or glass bottled juice without sugar
Rich and creamy cheeses	Cottage, ricotta, or hard cheeses
Fried and highly seasoned food	Tofu or bean curd, bean and alfalfa sprouts
Pickled foods only in moderation	Fresh fruit and vegetables
Coffee or tea in strict moderation	Herbal teas
All foods with added chemicals in strict moderation	

There are lots of good cookbooks that feature whole foods, and a number of writers have designed simple healthy recipes for busy people who do not have time to fuss. A parting piece of advice: beware of being faddy, fearful, fanatical, or foolish about food.

Contact Names and Areas for Teachers and Healers

International Network of Esoteric Healing

Australia

Judy Jacka
4 Joseph Court
Park Orchards, Victoria 3114
Ph. 03 9876 4774
judyjacka@bigpond.com

Harry Milton
2 MacGrath Avenue
5 Dock, New South Wales 2046
Ph. 02 9713 8041

Margaret Tapper
9 Macfarlan Place
Latham, ACT 2615
Ph. 02 6254 9348

Canada

Carol Martin
20 Poyntz Street
Barrie, Ont. Canada
L4M 3N9
Ph. 705 734 0107
clmartin@look.ca

Don Nichol
10 Essex Street
Toronto, Ont. Canada M6G IT3
Ph. 416 534 7024
donnichol@sympatico.ca

Czech Republic

Lucia & Ludger Scholl
Vinicna Alej 986
CR-252 29
Karlik
Ph./Fax. 42029912553
Ludger@ineh.de

Germany

Sybille Aston
Kurt Schumaker str. 8, 51427
Bergisch Gladbach
Ph. 02204 61160
sybille@ineh.de

Theodor Foemella
Ostereude 74
D-25813, Hussum
Ph. 49 484 183 8338
thformella@aol.com

Greece

Lena Livaditi
Kirkis St. 9
N Vousas 19009
Attiki
Ph. 30 1618 2110

Dimitri and Eri Tsinganis
Trivonianou 29
11636 Mets. Athens
Ph. 1698 4110
eridim@hol.gr

Hong Kong

Juilia C. McKenzie
Vitality Center
801Commercial House
35 Queens Road
Central Hong Kong
Ph. 852 2537 1118
health@vitalitycenter.com.hk

Netherlands

Elleke van Kraalingen
Wandelmeet 67
1218 CR Hilversum
Ph. 356 939 770
e.m.van.kraalingen@planet.nl

New Zealand

Lanie Murphy
44 The Parade
Paekakariki, Kapiti Coast, Wellington
Ph. 4 905 8021
lanilsphere@yahoo.com

Poland

Zuzanna Pedzich
UI Franciszzkanska 7/23
Warsawa 00233
Ph. 226 357 226

United Kingdom

INEH Teacher Group: The Hayloft
Palmers Green
Emsworth, Hampshire, PO10 7DL
Ph. 01 243 370021
Fax 01 243 431962

Helen Frankland
27 South Road
Chorleywood, Herts, WD3 4AS
www.ineh.org

Wendy Hewlett
47A Speldhurst Road
London W4 IBX
Ph. 20 8994 8653
whewlett@heist.tv

Dinah Lawson (see INEH Teachers Group)

Helen Loxton
5 Northville House
Northville Road

Kingsbridge, South Devon, TQ7 IAZ
Ph. 01 548 854028
theloxtons@onetel.net.uk

United States of America

Website:www.esoterichealing.com

Barbara Briner
3991 Shoals Drive
Okemos, MI 48864
Ph. 517 349 7377
b.j.briner@msn.com

Karen Disbrow
380 S. Treston Lane
Tucson, AZ 85711
Ph. 520 519 0536
azeteacher@msn.com

Wendy Glaubitz
7200 Noland Road
Falls Church, VA 22042
Ph. 703 560 8319
wendy1@ix.netcom.com

Deborah Graham
PO Box 518
Haslett, MI 48840
Ph. 517 333 8662
deegram123@aol.com

Martha Henry-Macdonald
135 South Street
Medfield, MA 02052
Ph. 508 359 2660
mhenrymac@yahoo.com

Margaret McRaith
5348 15th Avenue South

Minneapolis, MN 55417
Ph. 612 825 0111
pefMcR@aol.com

Julia Moses
3264 Bay Road
South Drive, IN 46240
Ph. 317 576 0588
julia@mergingminds.com

Rumiel Rothschild
41-610 NoNokio Street
Waimanalo, HI 96795
Ph. 831 464 4564
rumieir@aol.com

Tom Shaver
DO. 3075 Ala Poha Pl. # 1802
Honolulu, HI 96818
Ph./Fax. 808 840 1844
tshaverdo@netscape.net

Stan Shenefelt
7003 E. 85th Terrace
Kansas City, MO 64138
Ph. 816 356 6775
kchealer@juno.com

Zimbabwe

Adele Smith
24 Hopley Avenue
Greedale, Harare, Zimbabwe
Ph. 263 4 492181

References

1. MacLennan, A. H., Wilson, D. H., Taylor, A. W., Prevalence and cost of alternative medicine in Australia. *The Lancet.* March 2, 347:569-573.

2. Carson, R., *Silent Spring*, New York, Crest, 1964.

3. Tseng, R., Mellon, J., Bammer, K., The relationship between nutrition and student achievement, behaviour, and health—a review of the literature. California State Department of Education, 1980; and Serra-Majem, L., Vitamin and mineral intakes in European children. Is food fortification needed? *Public Health Nutrition*, 2001 Feb; 4(1A): 101-7.

4. National Health Strategy 1992: Issues in pharmaceutical drug use in Australia. *Issues paper* No. 4.

5. Smith, C., Best, S., *Electromagnetic Man*, New York, St. Martin's Press, 1989, chap. 9.

6. Chapman, J. B., *The Biochemic Handbook*, Revised Ed. St Louis, Formur Inc. 1994.

7. Mount, J. L., *The Food and Health of Western Man*, Bucks, UK. Precision Press, 1979, chap. 1.

8. Balch, P. and J., *Prescription for Nutritional Healing*, 3rd Ed. New York, Avery, 2000.

9. Mills, S., *The Essential Book of Herbal Medicine*, New York, Penguin, 1993.

10. Vithoulkas, G., *The Science of Homeopathy*, New York, Grove Press, 1980, chap. 9.

11. Wells, M., *The Bach Flower Remedies Today*, Melbourne, Autonomy Books, 1993.

12. Roth, B., Mindfulness-Based Stress Reduction in the Inner City. *Advances*, Vol. 13, No. 4, 1997.

13. Krishnamurti, J., *Commentaries on Living*, Third Series, Quest book, Theosophical Publishing House, Wheaton, Illinois, 1967.

14. Pert, C., *Molecules of Emotion*, New York, Scribner, 1997.

15. Tiller, W., *Science and Human Transformation*, Pavior, California, 1997, p. 55.

16. Burr, H. S., *Blueprint for Immortality*, London, Neville Spearman, 1968; Hunt V, *Infinite Mind* 2nd Ed., California, Malibu, 1996; Solomon J. and G. *Harry Oldfield's Invisible Universe*, London, Thorson's, 1998.

17. Tiller, W., *Science and Human Transformation*, California, Pavior, 1997, p. 127.

18. Oschman, J. L., *Energy Medicine*, New York, Churchhill Livingstone, 2000, p. 76.

19. Jacka, J., *The Vivaxis Connection*, Charlottesville, Virginia, Hampton Roads, 2000, p. 230.

20. Russek, L., and Schwartz, G., *Energy Cardiology: A Dynamical Energy Systems Approach for Integrating Conventional and Alternative Medicine*, Fall 1996, Vol. 12, No. 4, p. 4.

21. Dardik, I., *The Origin of Disease and Health—Heart Waves*, Cycles, Vol. 46, No. 3, 1996.

22. Maslow, A., *Religions, Values and Peak-Experiences*, New York, Viking Press, 1964.

23. Myss, C., *Anatomy of the Spirit*, New York, Bantam, 1996.

24. Ameisen, P., *Every Breath You Take*, Aukland, Tandem Press, 1997.

25. Bailey, A. A., *Esoteric Psychology*, London, Lucis Trust, 1942.

26. Steiner, R., *Introducing Anthroposophical Medicine*, New York, Anthroposophic Press, 1999, p. 65.

27. Wilbur, K., *A Brief History of Everything*, 2nd Ed. Boston, Shambhala, 2001.

28. Lucas, W. B., *Regression Therapy* Vol. 1. California, Deep Forest Press, 1992.

29. Bruce, R., *Astral Dynamics*, Charlottesville, Virginia, Hampton Roads, 1999, p. 119.

30. Jensen, B., *The Science and Practice of Iridology*, Escondido, Bernard Jensen Products, 1964.

31. Gorton, H. C., and Jarvis, K., The effectiveness of vitamin C in preventing and relieving the symptoms of virus induced respiratory infections. *J Manipulative Physiol Ther* 1999 Oct:22.

32. Grimm, W., and Muller, H. H., A randomised controlled trial of the effect of fluid extract of Echinacea Purpurae on the incidence and severity of colds and respiratory infections. *Am J. Med* 1999 Feb; 106 (2): 138-43.

33. Bailey, A. A., *Esoteric Healing*, London, Lucis Press, 1953, p. 156.

34. Fawsett, W. J., et al., Magnesium: physiology and pharmacology. *BJA* 1999: 83(2): 312-20.

35. Steiner, R., *Introducing Anthroposophical Medicine*, Hudson, Anthroposophic Press. 1999.

36. Holmes, M, et al., Impact factors on development of cirrhosis and subsequent hepatocellular carcinoma. *Compend. Contin. Edu. Dent.* 2001 July: 22(3): 19-33.

37. Mowrey, D. B., *Next Generation Herbal Medicine: Milk Thistle*, New Canaan, Connecticut, 1990, p. 108-126.

38. www.niddk.nih.gov/health/diabetes/pubs/afam.htm

39. Mingham, S. A., Diet and colorectal cancer prevention. *Biochem. Soc. Trans.* 2000 Feb; 28(2): 12-6.

40. Segasothy, M., Phillips, P. A., Vegetarian diet: panacea for modern lifestyle diseases? *QJM*, 1999 Sep; 92(9): 531-44.

41. Altura, B. M., Altura, B. T., Tension headaches and muscle tension; is there a role for magnesium. *Med. Hypothesis* 2001 Dec; 57(6): 705-13.

42. Lee, J., *What Your Doctor May Not Tell You About Menopause*, New York, Warner Books, 1996.

43. Kristel, et al., Vitamin and mineral supplement use is associated with reduced rate of prostate cancer. *Cancer Epidemiol. Biomarkers Prev.* 1999 Oct; 8(10): 887-92.

44. Anderson, J. L., The immune system and major depression. *Adv. Neuroimmunol.* 1996 (6): 119-129.

45. Baule, G. M., and McFee, R., Detection of the magnetic field of the heart. *American Heart Journal*, 1963 (66): 95-96.

46. Tiller, W., *Science and Human Transformation*, California, Pavior, 1997, p. 216.

47. Dardik, I., The origin of disease and health-heart waves, 1996. *Cycles*, vol. 46, 3. 67-75.

48. Barnes, et al., Impact of TM on CV function at rest and during acute stress in adolescents with high normal BP. *J. Psychosom. Res.* 2001, Oct; 54(4): 597-605.

49. Woolcock, A. J., et al., The burden of asthma in Australia. *Med. J. Aust.* 2001, Aug. 6; 175(3): 141-5.

50. Jacka, J., *The Vivaxis Connection*, Charlottesville, Virginia, Hampton Roads, 2000.

51. Becker, R., *Cross Currents*, Los Angeles, Jeremy Tarcher, 1990.

52. Gorton, H. C., and Jarvis, K., The effectiveness of vitamin C in preventing and relieving the symptoms of virus induced respiratory infections. *J Manipulative Physiol Ther* 1999 Oct:22.

53. Willard, T., *The Wild Rose Herbal*, Wild Rose College of Natural Healing, 1991, p. 56.

54. Lee, J., *What Your Doctor May Not Tell You About Menopause*, New York, Warner Books, 1996.

Index

abdominal pains, 92, 97, 108, 128
  case study, 127
  depression, 39
aberrant cells, 216, 240
Aborigines, xvii, 5
abscesses, 86-88, 127-128, 132
absenteeism, 91, 227, 286
acid,
  levels, 241
  overload, 96
  rain, 4
  waste, 56, 95, 156, 239
acidophilus, 113, 201
acne, 257
acupressure, 22
acute disease, 85-86, 88-89, 93
addictions, 5, 53, 117, 238
  traits, 239
additives, 4, 116
adenoids, 221
adhesions, 127-129, 142-144, 173
adrenal gland-stimulating hormone (ACTH), 60
adrenal triangle, 158-160, 287-288, 295
  See also triangles
  associations, 144
  balancing, 169
  case study using the, 120, 147, 153, 186
  visualizing the, 157
adrenalin, 57, 107, 141, 186, 190
adrenals, 47, 57-58, 140, 146, 211
AIDS, 46, 275-277
albumin, 116
alcohol, 18, 53, 69, 133-135, 301
alkaline/acid balance, 95
allergies, 141, 199, 231, 237
  case study, 92, 94, 230
  depression, 39
  food sensitivities and, 114-116, 196
  life threatening, 58
  migraines, 259
alta major center, 60
  case study, 276
  insomnia, 63
  location of, 265
aluminum, 12

Alzheimer's disease, 6
analgesics, 207
androgens, 58
anemia, 7, 47, 239-240
anesthesia,
  general, 266
angelica, 90, 109, 165, 260
anger,
  controlling, 119
  suppression of, 35, 89
anthroposophical medicine, 115, 308
antibiotics, 236, 240
  case study, 90, 193, 203, 233
  extended use of, 71
  overuse of, 7
antibodies,
  destructive, 126, 205, 211, 246
  immunization and, 224
  microzymal, 245
  production of, 111
  proliferation of, 115
  reactive, 116
  Rheumatoid Arthritis, 152
antidiuretic hormone, 58, 61
antigen, 174, 192
anti-inflammatory drugs, 147
anti-inflammatory herbs, 144
antioxidant, 17
  deficiency, 131
apple, 24, 95, 143, 197, 240
Arcane School, xx
arnica hypericum, 150
arsenic, 19
arteries, 35, 54, 183, 185, 189, 191
arthritis,
  blocked energy causing, 76-77
  forms of, 143
  inherited factors of, 143
  preventing, 141
  rheumatoid, 89, 141, 152-158, 193
  severe, 89, 99
asbestos, 227
aspartame, 131
aspartates, 268
asthma, 194-197

About the Author

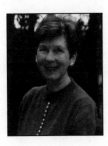

Judy Jacka, N.D., has been healing with natural therapies for more than thirty years and is the author of several books on natural therapies, theory, and practice. She has lectured and conducted workshops in Australia, New Zealand, England, and the United States. Jacka lives and practices just outside Melbourne, Australia.

Hampton Roads Publishing Company

. . . for the evolving human spirit

Hampton Roads Publishing Company
publishes books on a variety of subjects,
including metaphysics, health, visionary fiction,
and other related topics.

For a copy of our latest catalog, call toll-free
(800) 766-8009, or send your name and address to:

Hampton Roads Publishing Company, Inc.
1125 Stoney Ridge Road
Charlottesville, VA 22902

e-mail: hrpc@hrpub.com
www.hrpub.com